THE ALKALINE LIFE DIET

VOL. 2

FLIP MCGYVER

The trademarks that are used are without any consent, and the publication of the trademark is without permission or backing by the trademark owner. All trademarks and brands within this book are for clarifying purposes only and are the owned by the owners themselves, not affiliated with this document.

ent is geared towards providing exact and reliable information in regards to the topic and issue covered. The publication is sold with the idea that the publisher is not reQuired to render accounting, officially permitted, or otherwise, Qualified services. If advice is necessary, legal or professional, a practiced individual in the profession should be ordered. .

TABLE OF CONTENTS

INTRODUCTION..1

CHAPTER 1..3

Try The Alkaline Life Diet - Eating Alkaline Foods

CHAPTER 2..16

Choosing Alkaline Diets Is The Only Way To Live A Healthy Lifestyle

CHAPTER 3..20

What Are The Benefits Of Alkaline Diets?

CHAPTER 4..27

How To Get The Most Out Of An Alkaline Diet

CHAPTER 5..32

Top 10 Healthiest Alkaline Diet Foods

CHAPTER 6..38

Alkaline Diet - What You Should Know About Its Health Benefits

CHAPTER 7..43

Alkaline Health - The Benefits Of Following The Alkaline Diet

CHAPTER 8..49

Alkaline Diet Can Save Your Life

CHAPTER 9..54

Alkaline Body - Reach For The Ideal Body And Health

CHAPTER 10..60

How To Get An Alkaline Body Ph Balance

CHAPTER 11 63

Alkaline Diet And Cancer - Cancer Cells Cannot Live In An Alkaline Environment

CHAPTER 12 65

Alkaline Diet For Cancer Prevention

CHAPTER 13 71

Cancer Alkaline Diet For Survival

CHAPTER 14 78

Alkaline Diet For Dogs

CHAPTER 15 84

What Is An Alkaline Diet For Pets?

CHAPTER 16 88

The Best Diet If You Struggles With Silent Acid Reflux

CHAPTER 17 95

Alkaline Diet For Gerd

CHAPTER 18 102

Alkaline Diet For Gout

CHAPTER 19 106

The Alkaline Diet For Men's Health

CHAPTER 20 113

Alkaline Diets And Pregnancy: From Fertility To A Blissful Pregnancy

CONCLUSION 121

INTRODUCTION

THE ALKALINE LIFE DIET is a diet dependent on the consumption of ALKALINE FOODS, for example, fruits, vegetables, roots, and nuts, however, avoiding dairy, meat, grains, sugars and salts. Recently, this diet has been recommended worldwide by numerous nutritionists.

Whenever we digest food, it is either causes alkalinity or acidity. The two should share a certain balance. Sadly, the modern food that we eat is more acidic than it is alkaline.

Our blood must be slightly alkaline at all times. Whenever it shifts to acidic, this is when we experience a variety of health problems. These health problems are hypertension, heart problems, obesity, diabetes, and cancer. Every disease known to mankind is caused by acidity.

Today, there are many reasons why individuals indulge in the alkaline diet. Some use it as a preventive measure against diseases. Some use it as a cure for their condition. Some simply use it to lose the unwanted pounds. There is one thing that they have in common, and that is to get healthy.

This diet can do a lot for you. It can increase your energy levels; it prevents the production of mucus; it prevents and cures nasal congestion; it prevents and cures common illnesses such as influenza; it alleviates sensations like anxiety and irritability; it is a cure for and prevents chronic headaches, it prevents the recurrence of cancer, and it prevents the disease from ever happening.

As previously mentioned, fruits, vegetables, roots, and nuts are a part of the alkaline life diet. Dairy, meat, grains, sugars and salts become acidic after being processed by your body. Food is sorted as acid-producing or alkaline-producing depending on their pH (intensity of Hydrogen) values, where pH 0 - 6 is acidic, pH 8 - 14 is alkaline, and pH 7 is neutral (water).

To LIVE YOUR BEST LIFE I recommend you view your HEALTH, as YOUR WEALTH, this is the main reason a great deal of people nowadays are inclined to start alkaline food diets. Nutritionists worldwide agree alkaline diets are excellent for both your well-being and for your life in general. Alkaline diet foods are getting extremely popular among health-conscious people who understand their extraordinary health benefits. The blueprint for your ALKALINE LIFE DIET journey is all contained in this book…. THANK YOU for allowing me to show you how to LIVE YOUR BEST LIFE with the help of THE ALKALINE LIFE DIET VOL II. Enjoy!

CHAPTER 1

TRY THE ALKALINE LIFE DIET - EATING ALKALINE FOODS

What Is an Alkaline Diet?

An alkaline diet is essentially eating alkaline foods. The establishment for this diet is the high vegetable consumption. To get the best from this diet, we will give you some tips below.

Vegetables would be the most alkaline food around. Simple to purchase and simple to get ready.

Try to pick whole grain foods instead of prepared ones because handled items don't have the equivalent dietary substance. Some acidic foods, for example, limes, lemons, and grapefruits stay alkaline after absorption so are extremely valuable for seasoning.

Other acidic foods likewise processed in this diet are espresso, cola, and broccoli, artichoke, asparagus, beetroot, spinach, and cauliflower. Avocado, celery, garlic, ginger, onions, pumpkin are perfect vegetables to incorporate. Tomatoes, pears, papayas, mango, apricots, and apples can be incorporated. Nuts to utilize are sunflower seeds, almonds, and walnuts. Oats, dark-colored rice, and furthermore almond and darker rice, and also coconut and coconut water can likewise be utilized.

Its premise claims to be that one's diet may be able to change the pH value, or also the measurement of acidity and alkalinity of one's body. One's metabolism or the conversion of food specifically into energy gets compared to fire sometimes. You should know that each involves some chemical reaction which breaks down some solid mass. Nevertheless, the chemical reactions within the body occur in a slow moreover controlled manner. At the time that things burn, there is an ash residue which is left behind. The foods that one eats even leave an "ash" residue that is known as metabolic waste.

This metabolic waste may be alkaline, also known as neutral or acidic. The proponents of this diet say that metabolic waste may directly impact your body's acidity. Therefore, if you consume foods which leave acidic ash, this makes the blood more acidic. When you eat foods which leave alkaline ash, this makes the blood more alkaline.

Considering the acid-ash hypothesis, looking at acidic ash, this is said to make one vulnerable to illness plus disease, but alkaline ash is thought to be protective. If you select more alkaline foods, it is possible that you can "alkalize" the body and also improve health. The food components which leave acidic ash encompass a protein, phosphate as well as sulfur, whilst alkaline components encompass calcium, magnesium plus potassium.

Some food groups are thought to be acidic, alkaline and neutral:

- **Acidic-** This includes foods like meat, poultry, fish, alcohol, grains, dairy, as well as, eggs.
- **Neutral:** When looking at this group the foods are natural fats, starches plus sugars.

- **Alkaline-** Foods include fruits, vegetables, legumes, plus nuts.

These diets tend to have been promoted by many doctors. They propose that diets like these are able to treat or also prevent cancer, heart disease, the low energy levels one has, along with other illnesses. The human blood gets balanced among pH 7.35 and 7.45 particularly by acid-base homeostasis mechanisms. The levels that are more than 7.45 are said to be alkalosis. Levels that are below 7.35 are referred to acidosis. These both are said to be potentially serious. The idea put forward is that these diets are able to substantially impact blood pH for the aim of treating different diseases is not properly supported by scientific research. It makes incorrect assumptions concerning how alkaline diets works which are contrary to the human physiology.

Diets that don't contain any meat, poultry, cheese, plus grains may be consumed to make one's urine be more alkaline (higher pH), the difficulties present in properly predicting the impacts of these diets has resulted in medications, instead of diet modifications, like the chosen technique of altering urine pH.

Foods to Avoid

Red meat, poultry, dairy items, and bubbly beverages are foods that are the hardest to process. Your kidneys need to take minerals which are indispensable for the body, similar to calcium and magnesium, from the bones to disintegrate the acid in these foods.

It is not necessarily the case that little amounts of the above can't be utilized to enhance and change up your suppers. You will before long acknowledge what you can and can't use, as your body will let you know.

Move towards this alkaline diet slowly. If you eat a lot of meats or love dairy foods like cheddar, it might be best to attempt an alkaline diet supper three times each week, to begin with, so your body does not go into a stun. Any diet must be added to your routine gradually, and once your body acknowledges the new foods being offered, it will thank you by looking and feeling better.

THE REGULAR pH LEVELS PRESENT IN THE BODY

While talking about at the alkaline diet, one has to comprehend pH. Looking at it simply, pH is regarded as a measurement that looks at how acidic or maybe how alkaline something actually is. pH value will range from 0 going to 14 like:

- **Acidic-** 0.0-6.9, or

- **Neutral-** 7.0, or

- **Alkaline (or even basic)-** 7.1-14.0

The supporters of this particular diet say that individuals monitor the pH precisely of their urine. This is to make sure that it is alkaline (above 7) and will not be acidic (less than 7). Nevertheless, it is necessary to remember that pH changes much within the body. There are some areas that are acidic, and others that are alkaline. In fact, it is said that there is no particular set level.

The stomach is loaded with something called hydrochloric acid, allowing it to have a pH of 2-3.5. This is said to be really acidic. This acidity will be required to break down food. Whereas human blood tends to always be slightly alkaline. It has a pH that is of 7.36-7.44. When the blood pH is such that it falls out of the proper and normal range, it can be fatal when left untreated. But this only occurs during some disease states, like ketoacidosis that is caused by diabetes, alcohol intake and starvation. It does not have much to do with one's diet.

THE ALKALINE DIET MYTH

The alkaline diet; it is based on the possibility that the foods you eat cause a residue buildup after they have been used. This residue can be acid or alkaline.

These diets guarantee that specific foods can influence the acidity and alkalinity of organic liquids, including urine and blood. You eat foods with acidic residue; they make the body acidic. If you eat foods with alkaline residue, they make the body alkaline.

The acid residue is thought to make you weak against sicknesses, for example, cancer, osteoporosis, and muscle wasting, while alkaline residue is viewed as defensive. To ensure you remain alkaline, it is prescribed that you monitor your urine utilizing helpful pH test strips.

For individuals who don't wholly comprehend human physiology and are not nourishment specialists, diet claims like this sound not convincing. The following article will expose this fantasy and clear up some misconception concerning the alkaline diet. It is essential to understand the significance of the pH level.

Say, the pH level is a proportion of how acidic or alkaline something is. The pH level ranges from 0 - 14.

0-7 is acidic

Seven is neutral

7-14 is alkaline

For instance, the stomach is stacked with profoundly acidic hydrochloric acid, pH level somewhere in the range of 2 and 3.5. The acidity helps eliminate germs and digests food.

Then again, the human blood is marginally alkaline, with a pH of between 7.35 and 7.45. Typically, the body has a few powerful components (talked about it later) to keep the blood pH inside these ranges. Drop out of it is intense and can be deadly.

Impacts of Food on Urine and Blood pH

Food returns an acid or alkaline residue. The acid residue contains phosphate and sulfur. The alkaline residue contains calcium, magnesium, and potassium.

Food groups are viewed as acidic, impartial, or alkaline.

Acidic: Meat, angle, dairy, eggs, grains, and liquor.

Neutral: Fats, starches, and sugars.

Alkaline: Fruits, vegetables, nuts, and vegetables.

Urine pH.

The food you eat changes the pH of your urine. You have a green smoothie for breakfast, urine, in a couple of hours, will be more alkaline than if you had bacon and eggs.

For somebody on an alkaline diet, urine pH can be effectively be checked and may even give moment satisfaction. Tragically, urine pH is neither a good indicator of the general pH of the body nor is it a good indicator of general health.

Blood pH.

Foods you eat don't change your blood pH. When you eat something with an acid residue like protein, the acids created are immediately destroyed by bicarbonate ions in the blood. This response produces carbon dioxide, which is breathed out through the lungs, and salts, which are discharged by the kidneys in your urine.

Amid the procedure of discharge, the kidneys deliver new bicarbonate ions, which come back to the blood to supplant the bicarbonate that was at first used to remove the acid. This creates a reasonable cycle in which the body can keep up the pH of the blood inside a tight range.

In this manner, as long as your kidneys are working typically, your blood pH won't be affected by the foods you eat, regardless of whether they are acidic or alkaline. The case that eating alkaline foods will make your body or blood pH increasingly caustic isn't valid.

Acidic Diet and Cancer

The individuals who advocate an alkaline diet guarantee that it can fix cancer since cancer can develop in an acidic environment. By eating an alkaline diet, cancer cells can't develop.

This theory is exceptionally wrong. Cancer is able to spread in an alkaline environment. Cancer develops in normal body tissue which has a marginally alkaline pH of 7.4. Numerous analyses have affirmed this by effectively growing cancer cells in a chemical environment.

Cancer cells do become quicker with acidity. When a tumor begins to develop, it creates its very own acidic environment by separating glucose and diminishing flow. Subsequently, it isn't the acidic environment that causes cancer yet cancer that causes the acidic environment.

Considerably all the more intriguing is a recent report by the National Cancer Institute which utilizes nutrient C (ascorbic acid) to treat cancer. They found that by managing pharmacologic portions intravenously, ascorbic acid effectively destroyed cancer cells without hurting ordinary cells. This is another case of cancer cells being powerless against acidity, instead of alkalinity.

There are no logical connections between eating an acidic diet and cancer. Cancer cells can develop in both acidic and alkaline environments.

Acidic Diet And Osteoporosis

Osteoporosis is a progressive bone disease portrayed by a decline in bone mineral substance, prompting brought down bone thickness and quality and higher danger of a broken bone.

This is most common in postmenopausal ladies. It can really increase the risk of fractures. This theory states that acid-forming diets, like the standard Western one, will lead to a loss within bone mineral density. Known as the "acid-ash hypothesis of osteoporosis." this theory has its assumptions. Nevertheless, this theory does not consider the function of one's kidneys, that is vital in removing acids as well as regulating body pH. Our kidneys are able to produce bicarbonate ions which neutralize acids within the blood, enabling the body to closely handle blood pH.

Defenders of the alkaline diet trust that to keep up a steady blood pH, the body takes soluble minerals like calcium from the bones to remove the acids from an acidic diet. As talked about earlier, this is by no means evident. The kidneys and the respiratory frameworks are in charge of directing blood pH, not the bones.

The respiratory system is even involved in controlling the blood pH. At the time that bicarbonate ions from the kidneys bind to acids within the blood, they are able to form carbon dioxide that we breathe out plus water, that we take out as urine.

The acid-ash hypothesis even does not take into account a main driver of osteoporosis, i.e. a loss present in the protein collagen specifically from the bone. This loss of collagen tends to be strongly connected with low levels precisely of two acids. This includes orthosilicic acid plus ascorbic acid, or even vitamin C, in the diet.

You need to remember that scientific evidence connecting dietary acid to one's bone density or fracture threat is mixed. There are many observational studies which have found no link, whilst others have seen a huge link. Clinical trials, that are said to be more accurate, claim that acid-forming diets actually have no effect on calcium levels in the body. These diets are able to improve bone health. They do this by increasing calcium retention as well as activating the IGF-1 hormone that stimulates the repair of one's muscle along with the bone. Therefore a high-protein and acid-forming diet can be said to be likely linked to having better bone health, and not worse.

Although the evidence is mixed, most of the research present does not actually support the theory claiming that acid-forming diets will harm the bones. In fact protein, that is an acidic nutrient, seems to be helpful.

Numerous examinations have demonstrated that increasing animal protein consumption is good for bone digestion as it builds calcium maintenance and actuates IGF-1 (insulin-like development factor-1) that stimulates bone recovery. Accordingly, the theory that an acidic diet causes a bone loss isn't upheld by science.

Acidic Diet And Muscle Wasting

Supporters of the alkaline diet believe that to take-out abundance acid caused by acidic diets, the kidneys will take amino acids (building squares of protein) from muscle tissues, prompting muscle loss. The proposed system is like the one causing osteoporosis.

As talked about, blood pH is managed by the kidneys and the lungs, not the muscles. Consequently, acidic foods like meats, dairy, and eggs don't cause muscle loss. Indeed, they are complete dietary proteins that will bolster muscle fix and help avert muscle wasting.

What Did Our Ancestors Eat?

Various investigations have analyzed whether our pre-horticultural progenitors ate net acidic or net alkaline diets. Interestingly, they found that about portion of the seeker gatherers ate net acid-forming foods, while the other half ate net alkaline-forming diets.

Acid-forming diets were increasingly normal as individuals moved further north of the equator — the less accommodating the environment, the more the animal proteins they ate. In progressively tropical climates where foods grown from the ground were bounteous, their diet turned out to be increasingly alkaline.

From a developmental point of view, the hypothesis that acidic or protein-rich diets cause infections like cancer, osteoporosis, and muscle loss isn't substantial. Half of the Neanderthals were eating net acid-forming foods, yet, they had no proof of such degenerative disorders.

It is essential that there is no estimated fits-all diet that works for everybody, which is the reason Metabolic Inputting is so useful in deciding your ideal food. Because of our genetic differences, a few people will benefit from an acidic diet, approximately an alkaline diet, and some in the middle. Hence the truism: small time's food can be another man's toxin.

ALKALINE DIET - HOW DOES IT HELP?

Our blood has a pH somewhere in the range of 7.35 and 7.45, which is marginally alkaline. Alkaline diet depends on this pH level of our blood, and any diet that is high in acid-producing food will disorganize the parity. At the point when the body attempts to revive the balance of pH in the blood, the acidity of the food will add to the loss of essential minerals, for example, potassium, magnesium, calcium, and sodium. The imbalance will make people prone to sickness.

Sadly, Western diets are progressively acid-producing, and they devour minimal amounts of fruits and vegetables. Because of the approach of the alkaline diet, the standard of Western food has changed extensively.

Some diet and nourishment professionals trust that acid-producing diet may cause some chronic diseases and following side effects, for example,

- cerebral pain

- dormant

- visit influenza and chilly, and overabundance mucous generation

- uneasiness, anxiety

- polycystic ovaries

- ovarian pimples

Although some believe the above conditions are the aftereffect of acid-producing diet, and utilization of fruits and vegetables is gainful to wellbeing, a few specialists feel that acid-producing diet does not cause chronic infection. Other than that, there are proofs demonstrated that alkaline foods keep the development of calcium kidney stones, osteoporosis, and age-related muscle degeneration.

Neutral diet

Although an alkaline diet is favored, it isn't prescribed to have an unusual menu (eat all alkaline-producing food). It is more advantageous to keep a balanced ground of the two sorts of food. Merely make sure to observe the pointers above and counsel a professional/specialist before you attempt another diet.

If you found the above-mentioned tips valuable, visit weight reduction, diet and wellness experts for more information. To your dieting achievement!

CHAPTER 2

CHOOSING ALKALINE DIETS IS THE ONLY WAY TO LIVE A HEALTHY LIFESTYLE

The low starch and high protein diets doing the rounds nowadays are a solicitation to terrible health. All competitors realize that if a fit body is to be kept up one should avoid such foods. In addition to the fact that they result in extreme weariness are where weight executives are concerned. Choosing alkaline diets is the best way to carry on with a healthy life and additionally shed those additional pounds.

Citrus fruits, in general, are low in pH. These fruits are acidic in nature. The high quantity of citric acid leads to health issues including upper gastrointestinal problems, the formation of ulcers or silent reflux.

The acidic foods dissolve calcium in bones and teeth. So you should keep this in mind before drinking these highly acidic beverages direct from the glass. This is why it is important for you to use a straw before drinking citric fruit juices. Do not let these beverages come in direct contact with your teeth.

Fruits that don't intensify the upper digestive problems can be consumed on a regular basis for great health. These fruits are alkaline in nature and should be eaten every day to decreases the chances of the occurrence of chronic diseases. Majority of the fruits are alkalizing in nature, regardless of their initial acidic nature.

Alkaline diets expect one to pursue a balanced lifestyle containing the high protein low carb diets. The high protein diets leave the individual pursuing it exhausted and tired. It is for the individuals who have an inactive existence and need to shed some weight. Be that as it may, the pressure that is lost returns on when one stops the diet. With alkaline foods, this isn't the situation. The menus can be fused into one's lifestyle, and within days the results begin to appear. They expect one to eat around 80 % alkalizing foods to keep up the alkaline PH of the body to 7.4. High protein diets will, in general, make the PH of the body acidic instead of its regular alkaline tilt. At the point when the body PH ends up acidic, it draws in all diseases and drains one of energy. An acidic PH additionally results in fast degeneration of the human body cells. That prompts a shortened life. One should avoid these unhealthy diets and take a step towards accomplishing health and power by following alkaline foods.

Alkaline diets lead to the body pH keeping up its essential nature. The different body capacities are done easily, and the resistant arrangement of the body remains solid. Under these conditions, one feels active rather than feeling exhausted. Additionally, the weight shed like this stays off and above all the body does not fall debilitated. They help repulse illnesses rather than high protein diets which appear to draw in them. These designs are likewise useful for those experiencing incessant illnesses like joint pain, malignancy, headaches, sinusitis, and furthermore osteoporosis. Following such a routine while taking drug helps ward these ailments off from the root.

Alkaline water is additionally an absolute necessity for everybody needing to enhance their diet. No less than 6 - 8 glasses of salt-water can-do wonders for your body purifying. Processed food is all acidic and furthermore high on weight picking up substances thus ought to be kept away from. Drinks like soft drinks are highly acidic and ought not to be expended by any stretch of the imagination. It takes 32 glasses of water to balance-out one glass of soft drink.

Alkaline Water

Majority of the soda drinks and packaged fruit juices contain sugar in a very high quantity. In order to lead a healthy life, it's important for you to keep your body' pH balanced. The best way to do so is to keep your body hydrated with highly pure water. If you wish to lose weight, make sure to alkalize your body. Alkaline water is the best way to sustain the optimal pH of your body. If you want to shed a few pounds in a fraction of time, alkaline water is a healthier alternative.

How to shed weight by consuming a balanced diet?

Consuming foods rich in alkaline minerals is the best way to lose weight within the shortest period of time. In order to enjoy a balanced diet, you need to ditch the acid-rich food items. In order to consume a balanced diet, you need to identify which foods are acidic and which are alkaline. Once you understand the difference between alkaline and acidic diet, it will get a lot easier for you to achieve the ideal body weight.

Majority of the food items that we consumed are highly acidic in nature. Acidic food is responsible for excess weight gain in individuals. On the other hand, alkaline food helps to lose weight and allows the body to get rid of excessive harmful fat. This means the meal rich in alkaline mineral do not just reduce weight but also help in reducing the risk of heart attack and other cardiac disorders.

The balanced diet:

The balanced diet doesn't simple consists of alkaline foods. It's important to consume some acidic foods as well to balance the optimal pH ratio of the body. The optimal alkaline to acidic pH ratio of the blood is 80/20. Acidic food shouldn't entirely be excluded from the diet as some quantity is essential for the overall health of an individual. Majority of the nutritionists recommend consuming acidic foods in a limited quantity. A variety of acidic food items are high in their calorie count. But they are very nutritious when consumed in a controlled amount. In order to maintain good health, it's important to intake some healthy fats.

CHAPTER 3

WHAT ARE THE BENEFITS OF ALKALINE DIETS?

Ponder about the benefits of alkaline diets? At that point, you're not the only one, because numerous individuals would love to take in more about this good method for eating. This will help you bring in reality about what alkaline diets are and the points of interest that you can appreciate.

This nourishment program is called a few unique names, including the acid alkaline diet, the alkaline diet, and the alkaline fiery debris diet. These names all allude to similar fundamental ideas, which push fresh vegetables, fruits, entire grains, vegetables, and healthy oils.

Why the Interest in Alkaline Diets?

Researchers understand that the breakdown of foods results in side-effects that can be either acid or alkaline, and that these side-effects can impact acid-alkaline balance in the body. The perfect pH of a healthy body is marginally alkaline; however, the more acid-delivering foods that are presented, the more acidic the agency moves toward becoming. An acidic inside framework is in danger for various health issues.

An extraordinary lion's share of the foods that the ordinary individual eats today are highly processed, and they contain high levels of refined sugars, unhealthy fats, sodium, and synthetic compounds that add to health concerns.

Sweet moves, meats, and cream cheddar all deliver many acids when they are processed and assimilated. Processed foods are another kind of items that expansion the nearness of acidic mixes. These acids are immediately discharged into the body's circulatory system, which makes issues as the body battles to keep up its ordinarily alkaline pH balance.

Specialists say that you ought to have a pH level in the scope of 7.35 to 7.45, however, with the highly acidic American diet, it is hard to keep up a healthy pH level, as per alkaline diet specialists. These advocates trust that by supporting the body with the sort of diet for which it was planned, better health and longer life can be accomplished. People are worked for a menu of fresh deliver and other entire foods that have been exposed to insignificant handling.

What are the Benefits of Alkaline Diets?

As per sustenance specialists, it is an acidic diet that is at any rate somewhat in charge of fundamental issues, for example, untimely maturing and endless ailment. Health conditions, for example, joint pain and kidney stones are accepted to be connected to diets that are known to produce over the top measures of acids in the body.

Changing to a low-acid diet is accepted to be fit for expanding energy, decreasing bodily fluid, soothing manifestations of fractiousness and uneasiness, and may even prompt fewer migraines and diseases. Researchers are presently investigating cases that an alkaline diet can avert bone problems, muscle squandering, urinary tract issues, and kidney stones.

Ask individuals who pursue these diets, and they'll disclose to you that they're healthier, more joyful, and more active than their partners who continue all the more low-carb diets. A lot of individuals have discovered that their health issues have either diminished significantly or been entirely wipe out once they received alkaline diets. Shedding pounds is added an essential liven for the individuals who consolidate whole foods into their lifestyles.

Top 7 Alkaline Diet Benefits

The human body contains different processes and systems which interlock to make a machine which works with no glitches. Unfortunate diets and the ecosystem have to lead to the buildup of acids and acidic wastes in the body and different medical issues. These outcomes can be controlled and even diminished by following a basic diet plan for the accompanying seven benefits:

1. Weight reduction

This is the most significant benefit of an alkaline diet. With the regular western food and way of life including loads of acid-creating substances like dairy items and meats, and propensities like smoking, liquor, and utilization of medications, the body gets overwhelmed with acid wastes.

Acids eat and break down solid muscle, organs, and tissues. While fat cells shield organs from excess acids, excess body acids make fat cells protectively adhered to organs. When these excess acids are destroyed from the body, the fat cells are not required, and the body discharges them to incite weight reduction.

2. Oxidation

An acid build-up leads to the body cells not accepting adequate oxygen, which stops the cells' general functioning. Cells can die without sufficient oxygen; so expel acid build-up in the body by changing your diet and drinking alkaline water.

3. Mitigate sensitivities

Acidic environments exhaust the insusceptible system and take it into a 'reaction mode' wherein the body creates increased vulnerability to different things like substances, dust, and so on.

This is called sensitivities, and the body removes excessive poisons and acidic wastes through soreness, excess bodily fluid, swelling, and skin inflammation, which are altogether identified with hypersensitivities. The expulsion of excess acids from the body leads to the disappearing of sensitivities and related systems.

4. Decreased odds of treating degenerative diseases

The build-up of acid wastes in the body is the primary source for degenerative diseases including diabetes, kidney and liver disease, obesity, cardiovascular and neurological diseases, hormonal adjusts, premature aging and furthermore generally cancers. As neurodegenerative diseases flourish in acidic environments, the expulsion of this environment forbids them from increasing or creating.

5. Backs off the aging process

The buildup of acid wastes and breakdown of real capacities speeds up the aging process. A lot of body poisons leads to acidosis which discharges free radicals into the bloodstream, to assault and slaughter cell dividers and layers.

This leads to poor visual perception, age spots, weakness, poor memory, broken hormones, and other untimely aging signs. The expulsion of acids from the body utilizing alkaline foods counteracts further cell harm and switches the breakdown process.

Alkalizing diets are extremely important for the well-being of your skin. They contain a high amount of antioxidants. Antioxidants are extremely healthy for your skin. You can naturally consume these antioxidants by introducing alkalizing foods into your diet. These chemicals will keep your skin healthy and young. It will help fight the signs of aging. These antioxidants are so good for the skin that many skincare manufacturing companies add them to their skincare products. Antioxidants have no side effects. The best source for these antioxidants is fresh fruits, vegetables, and nuts.

6. Diminish blood pressure

Excess acidity stops the functioning of cells. The heart in this case works harder to make up for its languor, and this increases blood pressure. Also, high acidity levels lead to plaque build-up in the supply routes.

This lessens the blood vessels' thickness and increases blood pressure. So by expelling acidity in your system through an alkaline diet, you enhance your cell functioning and decrease your blood pressure.

7. Alkalizing diet for muscular strength

Acidic diet is extremely damaging to the muscles. On contrary, alkalizing foods help to strengthen the muscles and keep you healthy and active. Consuming alkaline diet alkalize your internal body environment. This neutral environment has an extremely positive effect on the body especially muscles.

It allows fast anaerobic metabolism. This means that your muscles heal quickly after a rigorous exercise.

On the other hand, people who consume acidic foods in excess find it hard even to carry their day to day tasks. They get extremely tired when they climb up the stairs or walk for long. This happens because lactic acid gets accumulated in their bodies when they perform a strenuous task. This acid stiffens their muscles and makes it hard for them to move their body freely. It gets hard for their system to provide enough oxygen to supplement all cells of the body.

In order to keep your muscles strong and healthy, you should embark on an alkaline diet. It will cure your stiffened muscles and will put your life back on the track.

8. Expanded energy levels

Acid builds up in the body brings down the body's regular adjusting systems as it leads to the siphoning of the more alkaline minerals like calcium, phosphates, and magnesium from the body's bones, tissues, and muscles.

Your blood in this way thinks that it's troublesome keeping up basic levels for ideal body functioning. This leads to drop-in body digestion, drowsiness, exhaustion, and even osteoporosis. Anyway, energy levels are expanded by reestablishing acid levels through legitimate diet and exercise.

By following an alkaline diet for its numerous benefits, your body is freed of amassed acidic wastes, well-being is kept up and various diseases forestalled.

9. Reduce the chances of a heart attack

Consuming acidic food is one of the major causes of heart attack. The body deposits extra fat in the arteries in order to avoid fatal leaks. This deposition or plaque constricts the arteries. This lowers the flow of blood within the arteries. When your heart is not supplied with enough oxygen, it gets exhausting. When your heart gets completely fatigued, it results in a heart attack.

Consuming alkalizing foods ensures a healthy supply of blood to heart as it doesn't result in constricting the arteries. This means that the chances of getting a heart attack are low. Balance your life by balancing the pH of your body. Start consuming alkalizing diet today. It does wonders for your overall health.

10. Benefits for the excretory System:

Alkalizing diets are extremely beneficial for the excretory system. It's important to balance the pH of the organs of the excretory system in order to keep your system healthy. Alkalizing diets are extremely important for the well-being of your kidneys. Alkalizing diets reduce the risk of the formation of the kidney stones. Kidneys are responsible to perform various purification and filtration processes for the body. If their health gets compromised, it leads to kidney failure. Kidney failure can be extremely fatal for your health.

In order to keep them healthy, make sure to consume less acidic diet and high quantities of alkalizing foods.

CHAPTER 4

HOW TO GET THE MOST OUT OF AN ALKALINE DIET

It very well may be useful to talk about to neglect of specific foods, however for the most part you should endeavor to eat a lot of fresh fruits and vegetables consistently. Plates of mixed greens are dependably a decent decision. Make a point to drink heaps of water, vegetable juice, or natural teas. Maintain a strategic distance from processed foods, singed foods, chocolates, foods that contain included sugars, and low-quality nourishment. Rather than adding sugar or salt to the meals you cook, have a go at utilizing healthy and tasty herbs and flavors. To wrap things up, remember that if you overcook your foods, you will lose a significant part of the dietary benefit.

Choosing a Proper Alkaline Diet Menu

Assembling a fruitful alkaline diet requires consuming the best possible foods and in the correct amounts. Your alkaline diet menu is urgent to the diet's prosperity. In this book, you will find out why alkaline diets are gainful to our health, how you can effectively execute your diet, and which foods you should put on your alkaline diet menu.

There are several protocols that nutritionists offer to the people who wish to balance their life by balancing their body's pH. However, it should be kept in mind that not every protocol works for everyone. In order to achieve the ideal overall health, it's important for you to get yourself tested first. Show your test results to the physician. Once he/she studies your condition, he/she would be able to provide you with the best insight of your condition. This will help him/her design a protocol specific to the needs of your body. When you get a diet plan customized to your body needs, you will achieve your ideal body weight and skin in no time.

Human Diet

Early man's diet was far not quite the same as what we expend today. An average human diet today comprises of substantially more animal proteins. Likewise, we currently eat a lot of highly processed and unnatural foods, which are loaded up with unsafe poisons to the body. Unreasonable salts, artificial sugars, and added substances increment the acidity of our modern diets. This expanded admission of acid removes the organization from its average, healthy, pH balance of 7.3, and damages to some of the body's necessary procedures.

In order to sustain the body's optimal pH; it's important for you to consume more plant-based proteins and fewer animal proteins. Plant-based proteins contain a high ratio of alkalizing minerals. These mineral keep your body in its natural balance. On the other hand, the animal proteins fall more on the acidic side. They result in the deposition of unnecessary body fat.

To achieve the ideal overall health, you must intake lots of fruits and vegetables. You should reduce the consumption of processed bakery items and carbonated drinks. Replace processed food with natural food items. Consult your nutritionist and discuss your ideal body weight. He will put together the perfect diet plan for you that caters all your bodily requirements.

How Alkaline Diets Work

By deliberately controlling the acid to alkaline balance in your body, you can benefit from an extensive variety of health benefits. Prolonged energy and weight problems will be promptly recognizable to somebody who is returning to balance from an excessively acidic body. By making your diet out of roughly 75% alkaline foods and just 25% acidic foods, you can restore your body to its healthy, common state. Likewise, setting up acidic foods with alkaline water can significantly diminish their acidifying influence on the body — an alkaline diet attempts to reduce the pressure set on your liver, kidneys, and different organs by having an excessively acidic (lethal) form.

Your Alkaline Diet Menu

The following are arrangements of various foods which are our best suggestions for having an alkaline diet. While foods which are acidic must be ingested for a healthy diet, they are too be brought down to the levels which our bodies initially adjusted to.

Alkaline Fruits:

Apples

Bananas

Blackberries

Dates

Oranges

Pineapple

Raisins

Alkaline Vegetables:

Broccoli

Cabbage

Carrots

Cauliflower

Celery

Eggplant

Mushrooms

Squash

Turnips

Acidic foods should make up close to 25% of your diet. Stated underneath are the kinds of food which are acidic. Remember that each class marked underneath has foods which are horrendously acidic yet also some who are considerably more on the alkaline side.

Acidic Foods:

meat

cheddar

vegetables

grains

nuts

select fruits

select vegetables.

CHAPTER 5

TOP 10 HEALTHIEST ALKALINE DIET FOODS

Have you ever heard about alkaline diet foods? If not, it's about time that you do. Work weight, homemaking, keeping up close to home and expert relations is inflicting significant damage on everybody's food habits, bringing about over 70% of the present age experiencing acidity and indigestion. Each third individual is by all accounts contracting gastric problems, heartburn, and acid reflux. The majority of this is because of the irregularity in the acid-alkaline pH of foods that expended nowadays, where you grab a snack and head to work. Fast foods, soft drinks and such are being consumed by youngsters, in this manner, it leads to inadequacy in minerals, nutrients, and sustenance.

Alkaline diets have been observed to be extremely beneficial for ideal health. You can avoid persistent ailments, for example, acidity, osteoporosis, and summed up shortcoming at a manageable distance with foods rich in alkaline content. Alkaline foods are vital since the pH of human blood is marginally progressively alkaline. This makes it essential that we have a more significant amount of alkaline pH than acidic content in the body.

What are the benefits of Alkaline Diets?

Alkaline diet foods have plenty of benefits, for example,

Enhanced obstruction

Energetic disposition

Expanded Alertness

Solid teeth and Bones

Simple Digestion

Alkaline diet foods are indispensable to keep up the pH levels of blood at an ideal of 7. Alkaline foods are for the most part vegetarian foods comprising of whole grains and vegetables.

Discussed below are the major healthiest alkaline foods for nourishing benefit:

Spinach and Greens - Spinach has been found to contain the best nutrients and is highly soluble. It very well may be eaten raw or mildly cooked. Other verdant green vegetables, for example, lettuce, fenugreek leaves, basil and so on likewise are incredibly high in alkaline content. They also contain a ton of minerals and nutrients as an additional favorable position.

Beet Greens – Beet greens may not be a very popular green present in the diet, its high alkalinity score allows it to be a good addition that one can put in smoothies and stir-fries. Beet greens even have a bitter quality which may aid in stimulating bile formation to aid in better-digesting fats. Beet greens are able to replace any green present in salads, soups, and smoothies.

Kale – Kale tends to be labeled as the new beef by some people. This is because it is said to be high when it comes to planting iron, calcium along with vitamin K, that claims to aid in keeping one safe from many kinds of cancers. If you have not tasted the kale, this possesses a mild taste which can enhance any recipe. Kale can be simply added to some smoothie recipe which requires greens, stir-fries, soups as well as salads for a helpful alkaline boost.

Swiss Chard – Swiss chard is a green which gives mega nutrition benefits. It has vitamins which support cellular health, like vitamin K. Looking at Swiss chard, this also has phosphorous plus plant protein. It claims to leave behind more necessary alkalizing minerals in comparison to acidity when metabolized. You can use Swiss chard like hearty lettuce wraps, within any recipe which has a grain bun or maybe tortilla.

Cucumber - Raw cucumber isn't just a zero-calorie vegetable, it is highly alkaline when eaten raw. It is heavenly and contains a large group of healthful benefits. Cucumber enhances by and considerable assimilation and keeps your skin fresh and shining. It provides healthy alkaline water that helps in flushing out undesirable toxins from the body.

Banana – Banana is one of the best foods due to its various dietary favorable benefits. It gives moment energy and is massively alkaline. Actually, on the contrary that you are experiencing extreme acidic problems, a banana diet can work wonders in reducing the strong sensation and heartburn amazingly. Bananas have fresh sugar content and can be eaten by anybody regardless of his health condition.

Bananas are said to be a wonderful source of fiber, that aid in promoting digestive regularity as well as sweeping toxins out of your gastrointestinal or GI tract. Some people may avoid consuming bananas so as to limit weight gain because of their high sugar content, but eating a banana is actually better in comparison to eating some granola bar and other processed food which contains much sugar along with acidifying ingredients.

Kiwi – Kiwi is another high-alkaline food. It also has a plethora of antioxidants, vitamins plus minerals. Kiwi is even a good source of fiber that can help with improved digestion, along with potassium needed for muscle function. Vitamin C is something else contained in kiwis.

Cherries – These are known as a good source of antioxidants like anthocyanins, that may aid in preventing cancer. Cherries are also said to help in relieving inflammation that is connected to joint pain as well as arthritis, moreover they may also prevent cardiovascular disease. You can blend cherries in smoothies.

Pears – This tasty fruit is high in fiber moreover lower in sugar. Therefore if you have blood sugar imbalances then this may be a fruit to try out. Pears have much of the antioxidant vitamin C that aids in protecting cells from carcinogens.

Celery - Celery is a delightful alkaline food that can help you tremendously in keeping your pH levels at the normal scope of 7. At the point when half-cooked, it gives greatest dietary benefit and can be eaten as the fresh plate of mixed greens as well. Celery also possesses additional cleansing properties. Due to the reason that it is mainly water, celery may easily aid the body in flushing toxins. You should also know that celery is regarded as a "negative calorie' food. This means that it takes more calories for one to chew and also digest in comparison to the complete amount of calories that it has. You can have celery in some green detox juice or smoothie recipe.

Broccoli - Broccoli is a standout amongst the most nutritious and alkaline foods that has substantiated itself over and over. It is effectively edible and is a rich source of essential minerals, for example, carotene and calcium. These minerals help in importantly enhancing resistance and battle diseases.

Avocado - This ponders natural product is a rich source of alkaline food and has a general benefit in keeping up great health. Avocado enhances your hemoglobin content and is extremely beneficial in reestablishing regularity in a disease influenced body.

Cauliflower – This is an alkaline food which can even help in hormone rebalancing at the time that the body's estrogen amounts are really high. This is due to the point that cauliflower has a nutrient known as Indole-3-Carbinol (or I3C) which aids your body in regulating estrogen levels. You may not have known this, but we have contact with estrogen daily via estrogenic foods (like soy), chemicals within the environment (like plastics) moreover pharmaceuticals drugs (like oral contraceptives). When you have high levels of estrogen, these are said to be harmful to your body and may result in weight gain, digestive symptoms like bloating, and reproductive cancers plus infertility.

Capsicum - Capsicum, otherwise called chime pepper is a rich enemy of oxidant and can be helpful whether eaten cooked or raw. It isn't just of high alkaline and health benefit, it is likewise extraordinarily delectable and adds taste to any dishes that are set up with capsicum for flavor.

Carrots – Carrots are said to be high-alkaline foods which are even known to improve eyesight based upon their vitamin A content. One cup consisting of carrots has above 300 percent of one's daily recommended intake specifically of beta-carotene, i.e. an antioxidant form precisely of vitamin A.

Looking at beta-carotene, this can even help protect one against cancer moreover help in promoting brighter and younger looking skin.

Potato Skin - Although potato is observed to be acidic, potato skin is exceptionally rich in alkali content. Raw potato juice is found to be extremely helpful in decreasing the acidic content in the stomach.

Sweet Potato – Although these are higher in starch, you should know that sweet potatoes claim to be an alkalizing food which gives the body much fiber, vitamins, along with minerals. Due to the fact that sweet potatoes are really high in fiber, they tend to have less of some negative effect upon blood sugar levels, as fiber aids in slowing the release of your sugar into your bloodstream. Sweet potatoes can, therefore, be said to be good food if you want to eat something for energy as well as for giving the body a boost of required alkaline nutrients.

Soybeans - Soybeans and soy milk are extraordinarily alkaline and can be utilized as healthful alkaline foods.

Hazelnuts – Most nuts actually have an acidifying impact. But this case is not present with hazelnuts. You can include these in your diet if you like nuts.

Cold Milk - Cold milk is found to have high alkaline content and is regularly prescribed to battle indigestion and acid reflux issue.

CHAPTER 6

ALKALINE DIET - WHAT YOU SHOULD KNOW ABOUT ITS HEALTH BENEFITS

Alkaline Diet - Take Alkaline Food for Better Health

The food that we take in today is different from our ancestors and ancestral diet was so different from what we are acquainted with nowadays. How appropriately said, "We are what we eat." With the headway of innovation, the types of foods we eat these days make us unhealthy. A view at the market will stun you with walkways and paths of handled food items and animal products. With the simple accessibility of fast foods nowadays, there is no trouble in discovering one in our neighborhood.

Craze diets are by and large halfway to fault for presenting radical new eating habits, this incorporate high-protein diets. Lately, utilization of animal products and refined food items have expanded as an ever-increasing number of individuals forget the daily supply of green foods in their diets.

It shocks no one why, nowadays, numerous individuals are experiencing unique types of afflictions and sensitivities, for example, bone diseases, heart problems, and innumerable others. Some health specialists interface these diseases in the kind of foods we eat. Particular types of food disturb the parity in our body that, amid such cases, health problems emerge. If no one but we could adjust our eating habits, it's impossible that aversion of diseases and reclamation of health can be accomplished.

Why Alkaline Is Important For Our Body

For a healthy body, the alkaline and acid apportion must be adjusted, which is estimated by the pH level in the body. pH values extend from 0 to 14 and seven is viewed as nonpartisan. Any amount under seven is considered to be acidic. Refined food, for example, meat and meat subordinates, pastries and some improved beverages generally produce an extraordinary measure of acid for the body.

Acidosis, an instance of the high level of acidic in the circulatory system and body cells is the primary record for the flow of various diseases delivering numerous individuals. Some health experts infer that acidosis is in charge of the underlying illnesses endured by multiple people nowadays.

Alkaline or alkaline diet, which regularly presents in our body kill the high level of acidic in the body to accomplish harmony state. This is the principle capacity of the alkaline in the body. Nonetheless, the nearness of the alkaline in the body is immediately exhausted because of the high level of acidic contents it needs to kill, and there is dry alkaline food eaten to recharge the problems alkaline.

The aim of having an alkaline diet claims to be to help your body maintain a good and normal pH, and not to increase your body's pH content. The things we eat influences the amount of compensating that the body has to do. Our body will generally maintain a pH that is of 7.35 always, but consuming acidic foods results in a burden. This is said to disrupt homeostasis. Consuming alkalizing foods is said to alleviate the stress present of long-term neutralization.

A Balance Alkaline-Acid Level For A Healthy Body

As depicted already, acidosis causes numerous health-related problems. Basic level of acid gets into our framework, breaking the cells and organs when not kill appropriately. To keep this, one must make sure that a parity pH is kept up.

To test whether our body contains a higher level of alkaline can be completed effortlessly. This with the utilization of pH strips which are reachable from any pharmacy. There are two types of pieces, one for the salvation and the other for the pee.

By and large, a spit pH level strip will decide the level of acid your body is delivering; the typical values ought to be somewhere in the range of 6.5 and 7.5 for the day. A pee pH level strip will demonstrate the level of acid; a typical perusing ought to be somewhere in the range of 6.0 and 6.5 in the first part of the day and somewhere in the field of 6.5 and 7.0 around evening time.

High Level of Acidity Is Harmful to the Body

You reliably experience the ill effects of weariness, cerebral pains and having ordinary regular cold and influenza; these manifestations demonstrate a high level of acid in the body. The impact of acidosis in the body not just restrains the common diseases that we know however different conditions that you may endure is caused by high level of acid in the body.

Wretchedness, high acidity, ulcer, dry skin, skin break out and overweight are a portion of those connected with extraordinary level of bitterness in our body. Not constraining to these, other primary and genuine diseases, for example, joint infections, osteoporosis, bronchitis, visit contaminations and heart diseases.

Indeed, even with meds, the manifestations might be camouflaged and keep on influencing your health as the foundation of the problem has not been entirely demolished. Taking more medication will aggravate the problem as the mitigating prescription will add to the acidic level in the body.

Alkaline Diet - A Sure Bet To A Healthy Body

To achieve the base of the diseases, our frameworks pH value must be kept up in a healthy state. Normally happening alkaline foods can enhance the lost alkaline levels in the body amid the killing procedure. By keeping up a healthy alkaline diet, adequate measure of alkaline are renewed in the framework accordingly taking shape back to the transcendent alkaline state.

So, what are the approaches to incorporate an alkaline diet into our eating habits? The simple essential initial step is to lessen the measure of refined food admission. As we know, these foods contain numerous synthetic substances which are the guilty parties in expanding the acidic level in our body. The subsequent stage is to eliminate the admission of meat and their subsidiaries and furthermore the measure of alcohol. The last advance is to expand the ratio of new foods grown from the ground, as they are generally high in alkalinity.

Oranges and lemons known for being acidic believer into alkaline after assimilation and consumed by the body is a decent alkaline diet. By and large, we should expend 75% of alkaline food day by day. The higher the measure of alkaline foods we put into our framework, the more noteworthy the balance of the acidic condition in our body.

ALKALINE HEALTH - THE BENEFITS OF FOLLOWING THE ALKALINE DIET

There are numerous benefits to following a diet high in alkalizing foods. One of them being that one gets a more significant amount of the vital nutrients and minerals your body needs in its characteristic shape which implies that it shows signs of improvement.

A diet high in alkalizing foods likewise implies that one has more energy to handle the everyday stresses and less dis-ease in numerous regards. On the Alkaline Diet, you may very well locate that a portion of the things that have upset you vanishes medium-term. Side effects like acid reflux, heartburn, IBS, hypersensitivities, feed fever, gout, joint pain, competitors foot, blockage and more can vanish truly medium-term on this diet.

To get the best benefits out of basic health, there are things that you can do to get progressively alkaline into your body, and certain things that you ought to avoid.

Things you should avoid if you need to get the most benefit out of the Alkaline diet is:

- Sodas - frosty beverages like Coke and different soft drinks are truly acidifying.

- Microwaved foods - the microwave changes the compound structure of any food you cook in it.

- Red meat - substitute red meat for fish or turkey and eat less frequently.

Things you ought to do to get more benefit out of the Alkaline Diet:

- Have the juice of a lemon or lime every day, one tablespoon full at once in a glass of water.

- Drink more water - no less than eight glasses per day.

- Eat increasingly green verdant vegetables - raw, cooked or steam singed.

- Add more flavors to your food, e.g., cinnamon, curry, ginger, garlic, cayenne pepper - these are magnificent for your health.

In any case, an expression of alert: like with everything else, one must not go over the edge. A few people new to the Alkaline Diet quickly begin overcompensating the alkalizing side of the diet. One needs to remember that you need to adhere to the 80/20 percent factor whereby you expend 80% alkalizing foods to 20% acidifying foods and except if you are engaging a disease, it is OK to stray off the diet now and again.

Having excessively of the one and excessively little of the other can lead towards disease, supposing that your body is too acidic you can end up wiped out, and if your body is too alkaline, you can likewise end up wiped out. So it is essential to expend foods from the two sides of the acid-alkaline outline!

HEALTH BENEFITS OF AN ALKALINE DIET AND EATING ALKALINE FOODS

An alkaline diet depends on standards of all-encompassing and Chinese medication, which have been utilized for a considerable length of time. An alkaline diet is roughly 75% alkaline foods and 25% acid foods. If the body is harmful, it can take energy and cause weariness, have poor processing, put on weight, have a throbbing painfulness, feel sick, and tired. An alkaline diet is a diet that accentuates, to a differing degree, fresh fruit, vegetables, roots and tubers, nuts, and vegetables.

Grains, angle, meat, poultry, shellfish, cheddar, drain, and salt all deliver acid. These foods imply that the regular Western diet is increasingly acid-delivering. An alkaline diet is a dubious dietary convention dependent on the utilization of for the most part fresh fruit, vegetables, roots and tubers, nuts, and plants and avoiding grains, dairy, meat, and overabundance salt, to balance the acidity and alkalinity of one's body. Clinical examinations demonstrate that alkaline water is the ideal approach to acquire alkaline minerals and acid rains like colas rapidly drain them. Our organs and organs work legitimately incorrect extent to the measure of alkaline and acid levels in our framework. Otto Warburg, a two-time Nobel Prize winner, these acidic and poisonous cells would then be able to wind up dangerous (he additionally expressed that these anaerobic malignant growth cells are crushed within sight of oxygen).

The most alkalizing type of foods is usually dark leafy green vegetables. This is mostly because of their high chlorophyll contact. At the time that you consume some acidic food, drinks and do little or no exercise, your body will need to function unnecessarily hard so as to maintain balance. At the time that it is functioning to restore equilibrium, your body will lose vital vitamins plus mineral. This offset is thought to actually increase the susceptibility that one has to disease plus illness.

The most alkaline diet is fruits and vegetables, and this is the reason a veggie lover and organic diet is compelling against numerous diseases. A vegan and organic diet not just underline foods that are alkaline, it additionally avoids the most acid-creating foods, creature proteins. This acid-alkaline balance is imperative since every real capacity, including breath, absorption, and digestion, work best at specific pH levels. The general proposal for lessening acidity by dietary means incorporates avoiding white bread, white sugar, refined oats, meat, angle, canned foods, tea, espresso, and toppings, while in the meantime expanding the utilization of fruits and vegetables.

Citrus fruits alkalinity affects the body and ought to be eaten to help control acid reflux. One quart of alkaline water expended 45 minutes before eating a dinner is ideal to assist in assimilation and avoid acid reflux or indigestion. Apples, mangoes, bananas, citrus fruits, and melons help keep up the body ph levels at 7. Alkaline foods are raw low-sugar vegetables, lemons and limes, grew vegetables and vegetables, and developed seeds and nuts.

The American Journal of Clinical Nutrition inferred that alkalizing diets enhance bone thickness and serum development hormone focuses; the acidosis is coming about because of acidic foods adds to bone and muscle problems. The hypothesis behind an alkaline diet is because our body's pH level is somewhat alkaline, with an ordinary scope of 7. The nourishment and healthy eating network have started to understand that what an individual put into their body can really affect how healthy they are generally speaking.

Cerebral pains, headaches, tension, misery, incessant weakness, asthma, obesity, coronary illness, malignant growth, ADD, chemical imbalance, and Alzheimer's everything conveys a shared factor: acid imbalance.

Alkaline diet and oral health:

Oral care is extremely important for your overall health. An unhealthy mouth can lead to a number of health issues. It can upset your stomach, cause ENT infections and disturb your digestive system. This means that your first and foremost concern should be your oral care.

Alkalizing diet can help you keep your mouth, teeth, and gums healthy. There are certain food items that you can consume to ensure better oral health. Foods less in their acidic ratio and high in their alkaline content are beneficial for your oral cavity. Hence they should be consumed more for improved oral health.

Incorporate neutralizing edibles and beverages to your diet in order to keep your dental cavity healthy. Eat alkaline mineral rich food like Soy including soybeans, miso, tofu, as well as tempeh. Make sure to consume unsweetened milk and yogurt. Add a variety of leafy green vegetables and fruits to your diet. Increase the intake of potatoes. Add herbs and spices to your meal. Limit the use of mustard, salt, and nutmeg in your meals. Add a variety of whole grains to your meals. Drink herbal tea for improved dental health. Replace trans-fatty oils with nut, seeds, avocado, and olive oils. Consume more seeds and lentils.

Calcium is not the only element that you need to keep your teeth strong and healthy. Other minerals are equally important to improve dental health. It's no secret that consuming calcium-rich products provide your teeth all the nutrients they require. You can supplement your teeth with calcium by consuming cheese, milk, and butter. You can also incorporate sea-food in your diet in order to ensure better dental health. Unsweetened yogurt is very beneficial for your oral health. If you are lactose intolerant then don't worry.

There are many other food items that can compensate your calcium requirement. These alkalizing foods include almonds and tofu.

Oral health is not all about in taking calcium. Other minerals such as phosphorous are equally important to alkalize your oral cavity. You can find phosphorous in red meat and pumpkins seeds. For people who are vegetarians, tofu is the best choice for alkalizing the body with the help of phosphorous.

CHAPTER 8

ALKALINE DIET CAN SAVE YOUR LIFE

The hypothesis behind the alkaline diet is that because the pH of our body is somewhat alkaline, with an ordinary scope of 7.36 to 7.44, our menu ought to mirror this, and furthermore be marginally alkaline. A lopsided diet high in acidic foods like animal protein, caffeine, sugar, and prepared foods will result in general bombshell this parity. It can exhaust the body of alkaline minerals, for example, sodium, potassium, magnesium, and calcium, making individuals defenseless against perpetual and degenerative diseases.

For the majority of us, living a balanced life is the foremost concern. However, balancing external factors like stress, personal life and work is not enough to lead a balanced life. It's important for you to have balance within your body. This balance is also referred to as "body pH". It's extremely important for a person to maintain balanced body pH to be healthy overall. This means achieving this balanced pH is one of the best balancing acts you can do for your body.

What's the Ideal pH Balance?

PH-balance is one of those terms that we get to hear a lot. However, only a few of us really understand what it actually is. Every Human being has two types of pH .i.e. an internal pH and an external pH. The internal pH means the body's internal pH. The external pH means the pH outside the body .i.e. the pH of the skin. The normal acidic pH of your body is 4 to 5.5. Conversely, the normal alkaline pH of your body ranges from 7.35 to 7.45. Your body operates its best within the optimal pH limit.

The alkaline diet theory:

According to the alkaline diet theory, every food item when digested has either an acidic or alkaline effect on our system. According to the research, acidic food creates the ground for the diseases to spread. The healthy diet should have 80/20 alkaline to acidic ratio. This ratio is what we call the optimal body pH.

The over-acidification of the body is the primary reason for all diseases. Soft drink is likely the most acidic food individuals expend at a pH of 2.5. Soft drink is multiple times more acidic than unbiased water and takes 32 glasses of impartial water to adjust a glass of soft drink.

Alkaline food and water ought to be eaten, to give supplements the body needs to kill acids and poisons from the blood, lymph, and tissues, and in the meantime, reinforces the robust and organ frameworks.

Most vegetables and organic products contain a higher measure of essential shaping components than different foods. The more prominent the ratios of green foods eaten in the diet, the more noteworthy the health benefits accomplished. These plant foods are purging and alkalizing to the body, while the refined and prepared foods can increment unhealthy levels of acidity and poisons.

Know that an excessive amount of alkaline can likewise hurt you. You should have the best possible learning of adjusting alkaline and acidic foods in your diet. After ingestion, alkaline food and water are very quickly destroyed by hydrochloric acid present in the stomach. The harmony among alkaline and acidic foods must be kept up altogether for your organs to perform well.

A healthy and adjusted diet is more alkaline than acid. In light of your blood classification, the menu ought to be comprised of 60 to 80% alkaline foods and 20 to 40% acidic foods. Regularly, the A and AB blood classifications require the most alkaline diet while the O and B blood classifications require increasingly animal products in their diet. Be that as it may, remember; in case you're in agony, you're acidic.

Progressing to an alkaline diet requires a move in one's disposition about food. It is useful to investigate new tastes and surfaces while rolling out little improvements and enhancing old habits.

Ancestral Diets and Acidity:

The examination of the acid-alkaline theory from the both scientific and evolutionary point of view reveals that around 87% of pre-agricultural humans consumed alkaline diets. It is believed that the idea of the modern alkaline diet originated way before we could even imagine.

On contrary, some of the studies suggest that 50% of the pre-agricultural human race depended on net alkaline-forming diets, while the rest consumed net acid-forming diets.

However, before believing any of these theories, it should be kept in mind that our remote ancestors belonged to extremely diverse climates with a huge variety of foods available. It is also believed that modern diseases would have been much less if our ancestors relied completely on alkaline rich diets.

Internal pH of the body

Our inward substance balance is mostly controlled by our lungs, kidneys, digestive organs, and skin. For important capacities to happen, our body must keep up an appropriate pH. The proportion of the acidity or alkalinity of a substance is called pH. Satisfactory alkaline stores are required for ideal modification of pH. The body needs oxygen, water, and acid-buffering minerals to achieve the pH-buffering while rapidly expelling waste products.

The external pH of the body

Skin is also known as the Integumentary System of the body. The external pH of the body is actually the pH of your skin. The external pH balance of the body is as important as its internal pH balance.

The imbalance in the internal pH affects the external pH of the body. This happens because the accumulation of the acids causes inflammation. As a consequence, your skin fails to act as a barrier against external harmful agents. This leads to the formation of lesions and sores. As a result, the open sores develop skin eruptions, redness, rashes and acne.

In order to keep your skin in its natural balance, it's important for you to improve your diet. The best way to ensure an ever glowing and healthy skin is to introduce alkaline food items in your diet. This diet helps you maintain the internal pH balance as well as the external pH balance. Everyone should embark on an alkaline diet to keep their skin and body young for long.

Alkaline foods are extremely important for optimal health. An alkaline diet strengthens your immune system. It promotes the growth of good intestinal bacteria and improves skin's health and tone.

According to some medical theories, kidneys and lungs are responsible for regulating the pH of the blood. They state that your diet doesn't play any role in balancing the blood pH. According to them the pH of the body remains the same regardless of the food we eat.

However, many studies reveal that consuming a low acidic diet helps to prevent the formation of kidney stones. The regular acidic food items we consume include meat and cheese. Replacing them with alkaline edibles like fruits and vegetables can help us maintain a healthy body pH. This type of food can help to keep the bone and muscles healthy and decrease the risk of type-2 diabetes as well as cancer.

Following an alkaline diet does wonders to your skin. People who follow an alkaline diet report clearer skin along with improved energy, stable mood, fat, and weight loss and a decrease in sugar craving. Alkaline diet simply doesn't balance the body's pH. It also provides us the essential vitamins and minerals that's keeps us active and going.

CHAPTER 9

ALKALINE BODY - REACH FOR THE IDEAL BODY AND HEALTH

Desiring to have the perfect body in part is less demanding than many people may think. At first, it appears to be anything but difficult to assume that changing to another method for eating is troublesome. However, despite what might be expected, the individuals who have attempted to consolidate the alkaline diet with their day by day life found that it's not troublesome at all and they can see the brilliant benefits.

In case you're somebody who has for quite some time been battling with a weight issue, finding a practical and compelling arrangement may appear to be an incredible thought. The individuals who attempted popular diets that advance eating just a single food aggregate experienced good pressure and torment, physically as well as rationally too. A portion of these accident diet programs helped them achieve the ideal weight however just for a brief timeframe.

The brief achievement of the diet program has caused dissatisfaction and disillusionment for some. Following quite a while of following a strenuous supper plan, they were at last ready to appreciate the aftereffects of their diligent work. The tragic thing is, the positive after effects of their dieting swung to be impermanent.

When they began eating foods that are not part of the diet plan, they started to recover every one of the pounds they lost. Far more detestable, they find that they are increasing more pounds that their different weight before they rehearsed the diet. You can envision how disappointing it is for somebody who has buckled down to acquire pointless outcomes.

Would we be able to anticipate a similar thing with the basic diet framework? You'll be happy to realize that accomplishing an alkaline body is something beyond achieving the ideal weight for your body fabricated. All the more critically, the basic framework is tied in with advancing by and large wellbeing, quality, and good health. For what reason would you be able to make sure that it's far not quite the same as other prevailing fashion diet programs?

The alkaline diet centers around keeping up a balance between our body's acid and alkaline condition. Reestablishing the body pH to its stability is the way to good health. Rehearsing this strategy of getting in shape gives you the opportunity to eat foods that are given essentially. What's more, nature has provided as a wealth of fruits, vegetables, and protein sources. We should recognize their alkalinity and acidity to accomplish balance and health.

Effect of the imbalanced pH on the body:

Digestive System:

Majority of the digestive disorders are the consequence of the excess acid present in the gastric region. These disorders include gastric reflux, nausea, indigestion and bloating. The pH of the digestive system gets disturbed when the intestinal tract doesn't have enough alkaline minerals. This results in the exhaustion of pancreases. This happens when our body is not supplemented with enzyme-rich food.

The lack of alkaline minerals makes your body lose its ability to process the food and distribute energy throughout the body. This results in a degenerative spiral of entropy in which organs get inflamed.

Circulatory System:

One of the principal causes of heart diseases is acidity. We all know that there are several fats that hold great importance for cardiac well-being. These fats are responsible for healing inflammation that becomes the cause of arteriosclerosis. Arteriosclerosis results when the arteries thicken and plaque are formed.

The major cause behind these thickened arteries is the excessively acidic internal environment. The accumulation of fatty acids in the arteries is actually the body's response to increased acidity. It lines the blood vessels in order to prevent fatal leaks which in turn cause imminent death.

However, this plaque also results in straining the heart as the aperture for the blood to flow gets narrowed. This exhausts the heart. Once your heart gets completely exhausted, you get a heart attack.

Immune System:

When the environment of your body is acidic, it serves as potentially great breeding ground for anaerobic bacteria. These bacteria are harmful to your health. The high levels of hydrogen in the body keep these pathogens inactive. As told by the great scientist Antoine Béchamp 'The germ is nothing, the terrain is everything.' The state of the bacteria depends on the pH ratio of the cell. This germ theory has helped current medical establishment a lot offering an insight into the cut, burn, and poison approach to illness.

However, radiation, surgery and pharmaceutical drugs offer an invasive approach. This invasive approach is not very useful as it doesn't work in the favor of body's natural functions to heal itself. This is why it fails to identify the underlying issues and only relieves the symptoms.

Respiratory System:

The transport of oxygen gets compromised when the tissues and organs are overloaded by acidity. When this happens the cells suffocate as they don't breathe properly. Each cell in our body requires to breathe properly. It cannot get rid of the acidic carbon-dioxide without proper gas exchange. When the level of carbon-dioxide gets higher in the cell, it leads to the formation of mucus and infections. These fluids and pathogens get accumulated in the lungs and result in colds, bronchitis, and asthma.

Skeletal System:

Arthritis is getting more and more common these days. It is becoming one of the most disabling diseases in developed countries. Arthritis means "joint inflammation". Arthritis is characterized by the swelling and stiffness of joints. There are two forms of arthritis namely Rheumatoid and Osteoarthritis. Both of these forms are associated with the pH imbalance in the body.

The joints get stiff when excess acid accumulates in them. The deposited acid damages the soft bone (cartilage). The cells produce synovial fluids and bursa fluids for lubrication. When these fluids get acidic, they cause dryness. This dryness results in irritation and inflammation of the joints.

When uric acid gets accumulated in the body it gets stored in the form of crystals similar to broken glass. It usually deposits in hands, feet, back, and knees. This condition is known as Osteoarthritis.

This condition is curable. You can use a specific protocol developed by experts using yoga and alkaline minerals.

Nervous System:

The excess of acid in the nervous system results in weakening of the brain. It deprives your brain of all its energy. This condition is also referred to as 'devitalizing' or 'enervation' of the nervous system. It makes the body physically, mentally, and emotionally weak.

Excretory System:

The excretory system is also known as the urinary system. There are several organs that join together to form the excretory system. One of these organs is kidneys. Kidneys are responsible for performing a variety of functions. These functions include the filtration of fluids and the purification of blood. If there is an excess of acids in the body then it starts its compensatory mechanism. It starts extracting the alkaline minerals out of the bones and dumps them off into the bloodstream. If this happens more often, kidney stones are formed that causes pain.

Muscular System:

Excessive acidity in the body damages muscles. This happens because the acids disrupt the metabolism of oxygen and glucose into energy. This leads to poor muscle performance in the acidic condition.

However, an alkaline environment ensures faster aerobic metabolism. This means that your body recovers from strenuous exercise at a much faster pace. People with acidic internal environment often breathe heavily while performing simple activities like talking to people and walking at a normal pace.

This shows that their body is in an acidic state. Your system finds it hard to supply adequate oxygen to all the cells of the body which is one of the most prominent symptoms of acidosis.

Reproductive System:

Not much research has been done to recognize the exact association between acidity and sexual dysfunction. There is still so much that we need to learn about how acidity affects an individual's fertility. However, health experts claim that acidity could be linked to three reproductive disorders including:

- The decrease in the sexual arousal in both male and female

- The decrease in female sexual enjoyment and orgasm

- The decrease in fertility and higher chances of miscarriage

CHAPTER 10

How To Get An Alkaline Body Ph Balance

The alkaline diet incline is quickly making up for lost time. Today numerous individuals from various spots comprehend the benefits of keeping up an alkaline body. An alkaline body is significantly less powerless to ailments than an acidic body is.

It is helpful to realize that a healthy life can be kept up just if one has an alkaline body. A touch of an activity routine alongside an alkaline diet will reflect in one's inward and external self. To accomplish an organization that is alkaline, it is vital that over 80% of our food intake establish of alkalizing foods. In any case, one should initially take the body ph test. It tends to be effortlessly tried using the spit test or the pee test. When the natural body ph is tilting towards the acidic side, prompt mediation is required. An investigate your diet will doubtlessly mirror an acidic pattern simply like your body ph. Social orders like America who live fundamentally on meats more awful still handled food are exceptionally inclined to losing the alkaline body ph. These sorts of foods have an acidifying impact on the body and cause a huge measure of harm to it. The American culture endures obesity as well as a lot of heart issues; this is because of their principally acidic diet.

There is a silver covering in this circumstance. A body ph in the alkaline range can be accomplished with only a little change in your diet plan.

Essentially put one ought to expend a lot of vegetables and natural products. A large portion of the acidic foods ought to be substituted by alkaline foods. A daily intake of around eight to ten glasses of water is an absolute requirement. Soft drink ought to be kept away from as is poison. Soft drink is very acidic, and it assumes control 30 glasses of water to balance on the acid in one glass of soft drink. A body that has an alkaline ph helps in switching the maturing procedure and furthermore keeping up a disease free body. The individuals who need to shed weight yet would prefer not to free energy should attempt alkaline diets and look and feel fit. The more significant part of other foods abandon one feeling depleted, and when one goes off the menu, the shed pounds is recaptured. In any case, trying to accomplish an alkaline body in addition to the fact that one feels fit and active the diet can be consolidated into turning into a lifestyle as opposed to an intensive lesson in appetite.

So get out there and check your body ph immediately. If you find that it adjusts from the normal alkaline body ph, change the manner in which you eat promptly. You will see that as your alkaline body ph comes back to typical, you will feel better from inside as well as sparkle on the outside. Your skin will feel more youthful, your hair will sparkle, and your nails won't be fragile anymore. A torpid feeling you felt throughout the day will be a relic of days gone by. So get out there and get an alkaline body and recover your young life once more.

Alkaline diet to achieve optimal body pH:

The foods that are alkaline in nature are potentially high in the essential vitamins and minerals required to keep the skin healthy and youthful. They contain certain antioxidants like beta-carotene, fatty acids, zinc, and vitamins C, E, & A, omega-3.

When you consume food rich in antioxidants, you protect your skin against skin cell damage resulting from the production of free radicals. These antioxidants are specially added to skincare products to keep your skin young and healthy. These chemical improve the appearance of your skin and reduce the signs of aging. This means that consuming alkaline diet regulates internal as well as external pH of your body.

In order to keep your skin fresh and healthy, you should consume lots of fruits and vegetables. You should add whole grains as well as ancient grains to your diet. These grains include amaranth and quinoa. Increase the use of good fats like avocado, coconut and olive oil. Eat lots of nuts and seeds.

Drink plenty of water. Make sure to drink 8-10 glass of water every day. Add herbal tea to your diet. Drink coconut water more often. Almond milk is also very good for the health of your skin. Mix apple cider vinegar with water and drink it on a regular basis. Green smoothies can also be consumed to regulate the external pH of the body.

There are certain foods that you should stop consuming altogether or at least reduce their use in your daily life. Make sure to consume red meat and chicken as less as you can. Don't intake processed food. Stop consuming biscuits, bread, and cake. Minimize the intake of soft drinks as they contain high levels of carbon dioxide. Decrease alcohol consumption. Reduce the intake of caffeinated food items like tea and coffee. Don't consume chocolates in excess.

CHAPTER 11

ALKALINE DIET AND CANCER - CANCER CELLS CANNOT LIVE IN AN ALKALINE ENVIRONMENT.

Ever asked why the heart never gets cancer. The core may get influenced inevitably by disease or some other piece of the body however we never know about cancers of the hearts. Cancer only occurs in those cells that have the tendency to duplicate or cause mutation, which ultimately passes to the daughter cells. As far as the heart is concerned, the heart cells do not duplicate or cause any mutation and they just keep pumping to regulate the blood circulation. This is one of the main reasons why the heart does not get cancer. The alkaline diet is maybe the main perpetual approach to avoid and free oneself of cancer.

Give us a chance to comprehend what causes cancer and how an alkaline diet can forestall it. Every cell in our body takes in oxygen, supplements, and glucose while tosses out poisons. The immune system ensures these cells. Be that as it may, as the body gets acidic the immune system gets overwhelmed by the toxins and the battery loses its ability to take in oxygen and accordingly matures. This cell gets cancer influenced and is lost. Cancers cells lie dormant in a ph of 7.4 yet as the body receives alkalized higher and the ph level achieves 8.4 these malignant cells cease to exist. So the response to cancer lies in a to a high degree alkaline diet. With the correct utilization prompting an upper alkaline body ph the cancer cells can't live in that condition and cease to exist.

Cancer cells being anaerobic can't live in oxygen. They can flourish in low oxygen conditions. At the point when the ph of the body is kept up by devouring an alkaline diet the immune system of the body remains solid. This prompts the cells getting enough oxygen and disposing of their poison squander. Cancer will neither flourish nor take birth under such conditions.

How does an alkaline diet avert cancer? Such a menu prompts a high alkaline body ph. This upper alkaline body ph results in alkaline tissues in the body. Alkaline tissues hold multiple times more oxygen than acidic tissues. Cancer can't live in an oxygenated atmosphere. If the cells are oxygen-rich, they will counteract cancer. In this manner, while an acidic mass will be a perfect ground for cancer to create and additionally spread, an alkaline mass will crush cancer cells. Having a lot of greens vegetable and fruit alongside alkaline water can spare you from cancers. To give your body the best alkaline/acidic parity expects one to eat foods that are exceedingly alkalizing while at the same time staying away from the acidifying foods.

CHAPTER 12

ALKALINE DIET FOR CANCER PREVENTION

Do you realize that Alkaline diet counteracts cancer? Indeed, some free radicals are caused by our very own food intake and various contaminations noticeable all around and water. The best thing we can do is changes our way of life and know about the food that we take in our body. Shockingly, western diet merely is ordinarily acidic. This surprises the balance of our internal territory and ecosystem that can cause a lot of diseases like cancer.

Cancer Facts

- It is possible to get a cure from cancer at in newly diagnosed people.

- Cancer is relatively more curable when it gets detected at early stages.

- Although it is observed in certain cases that cancer develops without too many symptoms in the body.

- But it is most likely that even when cancer shows some kind of symptoms in your body, you may overlook it thinking that it is not cancer. This is particularly devastating and very lethal.

How To Handle Cancer Symptoms At Its Early Stage?

As discussed earlier that cancer does not depict any symptoms especially at the early stage, it becomes very important for you to undergo cancer screening tests to minimize the risk factor as much as you can. Cancer is confined to certain age groups and your family doctor is the best judge to suggest you the screening test for the detection of cancer in your body.

People (who are smokers, genetics, take a heavy amount of alcohol, face direct sun exposure during their work etc.) having the risk factor of being involved in this disease must be accurately aware of the early symptoms. The only way to avoid this disease is to adopt precautionary measures.

Common Signs and Symptoms of Cancer

- When you feel a Constant cough or saliva observed with blood-tinged. These symptoms normally show common infections including bronchitis or sinusitis. Furthermore, these symptoms may be of the lungs, neck, and head.

- When you see some kind of change in your bowel habits. Bowel habits are mostly related diet and the fluid that you take in. When you suffer consistent diarrhea, this kind of symptoms usually lasts for weeks.

- When there is some kind of blood in the stool.

- When unexplained anemia is observed.

- Unusual enlargement in the breast.

- When there are lumps in the testicles.

- Unusual frequent urination which is uncontrollable.

As indicated by WHO, cancer is one of the primary sources of deaths on the planet. The uplifting news is, cancer can be forestalled. Before we get into counteractive action, let me clarify how the tumor is analyzed by revealing to you a portion of the symptoms. Note that symptoms may change from a case to case premise.

The most well-known symptoms of cancer are bumps, swelling, and dying. The pressure of surroundings organs may likewise cause jaundice. At whatever point you feel debilitated and tired it may be a case of persistent weakness, yet it might be caused by something unique inside and out. It is smarter to change to an alkaline diet to anticipate cancer. Shoddy nourishment and other "dead" foods can cause a lot of diseases in our body. It is smarter to know the distinction of the foodstuff that we put in our body.

You can begin changing your way of life by practicing or participating in physical exercises. You can detoxify your body by sweating it out. Couple your activity propensity with a balanced diet and you will see a distinction in your energy level and execution in your activity or at home.

Make sure to locate a fun exercise or game that will suit your enthusiasm for quite a while. Merely have a fabulous time and alkalize your diet. With an alkaline body, you will avert cancer extra time. To battle free radicals, attempt and be aware of your food intake. Stay away from low-quality nourishment and undesirable propensities like drinking and smoking. Trust me; you will be in an ideal situation without it.

On the off chance that you don't need an extreme change in the way of life, locate an alkaline diet system that is compelling for you. The best diet system can produce results in only three days. In the multi-week, the impacts will be full and finish. It appears to be staggering however it is valid, a lot of individuals who enhanced their lives as a result of this change in diet.

Why The Alkaline Diet And Cancer Is An Ideal Solution

Well, there is a strong relationship between the acidic environment and the cancer cells. Research has shown that the acidic environment allows the cancer cells to grow. So a diet which is high in alkaline nutriments means high in pH, and alkaline food which is comparatively low in acidic food is always going to raise the level of pH in the body. The rise in pH level means making someone's body more alkaline, can certainly not only prevent from cancer but also will cure against the cancer disease.

Because of the pandemic of cancer that has broken out as of late, there have been significant steps made in where cancer began, how it develops in the body and how alkaline diet and cancer routine has progressed toward becoming. The meaning of cancer enables the patient to have some control over the anticipation and skirmish of cancer cells. By adhering to a primarily alkaline diet, this diminishes, and indeed extinguishes, the generation of cancer and different diseases. Along these lines, an alkaline diet has been found to counteract illness, while an acidic food urges disease and cancer to develop.

When you take the meaning of cancer basically, it is 'a malformed cell.' This abnormal cell can duplicate abnormal cells, and since the human body repeats a vast number of cells day by day, the appropriate response is to stop that propagation. The best protection at that point is a decent offense, and that is the thing that an alkaline diet does as it encourages the great cells, while stifling out the disease.

The foods that are taken into the body usually originate from two classes - foods that deliver an acidic domain and foods that create an alkaline situation. If you are considering an extensive amount of meds, this may make your system lean more towards the acidic; however, it tends to be balanced by expending progressively alkaline-producing foods.

An alkaline diet is commonly comprised of alkaline-producing foods, with the goal that the pH level is conveyed to a level of around 7.4. You seek online there are alkaline/acidic outlines of the considerable number of foods. If you are merely starting this diet, duplicate the diagram and convey it with you when you shop or go out to eat. As a rule, avoid handled foods, fast foods browned in trans fat, any diet made with white sugar or white flour, and all foods with synthetic compounds and steroids. These foods all feed cancer cells. If this is the thing that your diet is comprised of, check the basic food rundown and see what to eat now.

Foods on that are alkaline-producing are vegetables, seeds, most organic products, darker rice and different grains, and fish. These foods can be blended and coordinated to your inclination for in any event 80% of your aggregate diet, and afterward, you include 20% of the acidic-producing foods, and the acidic foods are not all "awful." Meals on the acidic side are entire grain bread, lean meats, drain and drain items, margarine, and eggs, and this signifies to make a 100% alkaline diet.

To screen your pH level once you have begun on an alkaline diet and cancer battling method for eating, check any well-being food store for pH strips or litmus paper. There will be a shading outline included to utilize and figure out what your pH blood level is. For a primary system, it should enlist between 7.2 - 7.8. No two individuals are similar, so test your pH level about once per day as you begin. At that point keep on checking once every week. If you have to raise your pH level, eat increasingly alkaline foods and utilize green enhancements. An alkaline diet will avert disease usually.

Chapter 13

Cancer Alkaline Diet For Survival

Before going deep in into the detail, it is important to know that what actually alkaline diet is, and what is the purpose or role it plays in the body when it is taken.

The alkaline diet focuses around taking alkaline diet and fluids while minimizing or reducing the consumption of foods that result in the formation of acid in the body.

Now the question arises what are the acid forming foods? The answer is alcohol, fast foods, gluten, sugar, animal protein, sweets, takeaways, pastries, pasta and many more.

On the other what are the alkaline-forming foods? Again the answer is simple and clear, these include, greens, vegetables, fresh foods, oats, beans, pulses, veggies like spinach, broccoli, kale, coconut milk or oil, fish, nuts, fruits with low sugar, spices up to some extent, herbs and shrubs etc.

A cancer alkaline diet can give a stable hand on your shoulder with regards to keeping your body sound and lessening the danger of the assault and beginning of cancerous cells. At the point when a lot of acids is retained, processed and utilized into the body, it changes the ordinary pH equalization of your blood. Your blood is slightly alkaline commonly and on the off chance that, by the environment or foods changes to a progressively acidic nature, issues can emerge and the inward body can turn into a prime rearing ground for disease.

A decent, stable, adjusted cancer alkaline diet can help forestall not just gentle ailments extending from influenza to cerebral pains, yet also cancer. A cancer alkaline diet, substantial on vegetables, organic products, vegetables and seeds and so forth, merits considering safeguard measures.

Without the vital equalization of alkaline in your diet (alkaline originate from such sources as new foods grown from the ground), the body should discover approaches to manage the excess of acid that will be noticeable in your system. The body will move excess fat to someplace in the body, finding a dumping ground for all the excess so the blood will have the capacity to keep its common pH level of around 7.4 (alkaline). Be that as it may, it has needed to strive to arrive, and the more the body needs to dump this hazardous excess of acid, the regions where it is being saved will endure cell rot. It's an endless loop as then the dead cells will transform into acid as well, bringing on additional build up and poisons. The cells that do figure out how to make due through adjusting will do as such by getting to be 'outside' to the body, or dangerous. This is cancer.

Acidic foods incorporate things like meat, dairy, desserts, liquor, chocolate is regularly the sorts of foods that are taken in wealth over alkaline based ones. It has been recommended by research that a straightforward change in diet can help shield you from the danger of cancer. There are different benefits to changing to a cancer alkaline diet. Regardless of whether you are merely feeling kept running down, at that point primarily by changing what goes into your body, your fuel can bring benefits of enhancing your internal activities, as well as can give you the additional energy, imperativeness and help to get thinner. A body which is slightly alkaline can be imperative for keeping up great well-being for it advances great oxygenation in the blood. Cancer can't make due in all around oxygenated environments. It flourishes in low-oxygenated, consequently acidic, residences.

Different approaches to give your pH balance a lift is to clean up or expanding your breath rate and not to overcook vegetables which demolishes fundamental supplements. Boosting your admission and receiving the benefits of the majority of the integrity that Mother Nature put into her products of the soil, will lead you to a more useful life, help in the aversion of diseases and ailments and help keep you youthful and lively. Changing to a higher alkaline based diet can keep these cancerous cells framing.

HOW AN ALKALINE DIET CAN HELP FIGHT CANCER

Regardless of if you need to control the development of cancer in your body or are merely searching for a more advantageous diet, transforming from an acidic to alkaline lifestyle is essential for enhanced general wellbeing.

Typically, it isn't feasible for ailments to exist in an alkaline domain. This implies by adjusting your inward pH levels; you can restrict or control your weakness to illnesses. It likewise backs off the rate of free radicals and other hurtful impacts in the body. This is the premise of how an alkaline diet can help fight cancer.

1. Make it a point to drink however much water as could be expected because it is the best establishment of an all-alkaline diet. As alkaline platelets hold a most extreme of multiple times more oxygen than acidic cells, including

eight glasses of water to your day by day food and drink utilization makes a checked contrast in the measure of oxygen, your batteries can hold. Water positions around seven on the pH scale and can oxidize and sustain cells while flushing out every one of the poisons transmitted by acidic substances.

2. If you have been determined to have cancer, it is smarter to set present moment and long-haul diet objectives to graph your advancement. This is basic as you have to make an emotional move in your pH levels to fight cancer, by making whatever critical number changes to your body as would be prudent.

3. Diminish or quit devouring foods high in pH levels like espresso, fake sugars, dark tea, alcohol, hamburger, and pork (as all meats are acidic to some extent), prepared cheddar, over-handled foods, foods containing medications and added substances, peanuts, soft drinks, and white bread and rice. Likewise dodge all sugars and foods containing mostly hydrogenated oils, which is available in for all intents and purposes everything from solidified foods to cheddar items. It demonstrates accommodating to make a rundown of foods and drinks you generally devour and discover the acidic rating of every one of them.

4. This done, supplant acidic foods with more beneficial choices like eating whole grains rather than white foods and drinking herb teas and vegetable squeezes rather than soft drinks. Expand a more significant amount of raw vegetables, entire grains, yogurt, white potatoes, sweet potatoes, and beans. While a veggie lover diet is viewed as the best alternative for a high-alkaline balance, you can at times incorporate poached fish or naturally raised meat to your food.

5. Eat an all-around balanced diet of products of the soil. A few vegetables like the cruciferous assortment are full of supplements, as well as contain cancer-fighting mixes. Precedents are broccoli, cabbage, turnips, collards, kale, bok choy, cauliflower, Brussels sprouts, and arugula.

6. Studies performed by the National Cancer Institute a couple of years back referenced that 2 out of 3 cancer authorities recommended following a 70% homemade food diet while a little level of them favored after a half raw food diet.

Fight Cancer With the Alkaline Diet

Do you realize that global cancer rates could increment by half to 15 million by 2020? Cancer has been the primary source of death worldwide for quite a while. Cancer was mindful with 13% of passing comprehensively.

You can prevent cancer with alkaline diet and appropriate lifestyle far from different indecencies.

Tips to fight cancer

1. You can attempt and lift your safe framework so you can prevent cancer. One route is to take multivitamins and eat vegetables wealthy in supplements.

2. Take food rich in lycopene. Tomato-based dishes are an extraordinary wellspring of rich lycopene for your body.

3. See a specialist for regular registration. There are a lot of sorts of cancer that you won't have the capacity to distinguish with expert restorative help. So it's smarter to look for the assistance of your physician. Exploit your nearby medicinal administrations.

4. Stay far from alcohol and falsely seasoned foodstuffs to abstain from blocking your body with garbage and free radicals.

5. Stay far from consumed meat. However much as could be expected, eat vegetable dishes. It is nutritious, and it tastes extraordinary as well.

6. 6Try to eat a lot of fruits and vegetables. Vegetables and fruits are rich in vitamins and other nutrients that are resistant against diseases like cancer.

7. Take green tea in several intervals in your daily routine. Green tea has antioxidants in it, so by taking green tea several times in a day, it can certainly help you fight against the disease.

8. Going outside in sun heat is quite beneficial. Sunlight has the tendency to improve your overall mood, it creates optimism and helps your immune system to fight against the invaders and protects from causing cancer.

9. Increased use of Beta Glucans. Beta-glucans exist naturally but are not available in the human body. These are a kind of sugar molecules that aid the immune system in the body and cure against cancer. These Beta glucan can be extracted from mushrooms, yeast, fiber, oats, and barley.

Cancer and alkaline diet arrangement

You can evade cancer with alkaline diet and a couple of minor lifestyle changes. If you feel drowsy, tired, and debilitated constantly, have a go at changing your food admission. You will see the distinction in your body. You will get fit and feel more youthful and energetic. Your life will be vigorous and full of young essentialness.

Regardless of whether you don't presume you have cancer, the alkaline diet is an excellent answer for help you feel youthful and invert the maturing procedure. With the blend of a balanced diet and some everyday exercise routines, you'll feel distinctive by and large about your wellbeing. You will have a trim body in an about multi-month.

Attempt to be cancer free with the alkaline diet, or only feel solid and sound. Keep in mind that a marginally soluble body is significant for good wellbeing. Extremely acidic bodies are rich rearing reason for a lot of types of constant ailments. That is the reason you have to balance the pH of your body. Endeavor to alkalize your body with a decent diet to save yourself from passionate agony and budgetary misuse of a yo-yo diet.

Maintain a strategic distance from worry with a healthy lifestyle and a balanced diet. You don't need to break your old eating designs with an alkaline diet. You don't need to surrender drinking a jug or two. You should merely continue eating extra alkaline food.

CHAPTER 14

ALKALINE DIET FOR DOGS

Alkaline diet for the dog can change his health, and it might be encouraged to help lighten certain canine health conditions. How about we take a look at what pH levels mean, what the pH level of most industrially arranged dog foods are, the parts of an alkaline diet, how soluble water may encourage your dog, what health benefits alkaline diets or water give and if there are cases when they may not be a smart thought for your pet.

Before we examine the better purposes of an alkaline diet, how about, we take a couple of minutes to audit the distinction between alkaline and acidic pH. Arrangements are estimated on a scale from 0 to 14, and they are viewed as alkaline if their pH level is higher than 7. Provisions are viewed as acidic if their pH level measures beneath 7. Unadulterated water is considered to be impartial at the midpoint of the scale with a pH level of 7.

To the extent your dog's health is concerned, his blood or urinary pH levels might be talked about by your veterinarian. Urinary pH is of specific concern if your dog is inclined to kidney or bladder stone.

The pH Levels of Commercially Prepared Dog Foods

Normally the pH in dogs ranges from 5.5 to 7.0. But this range may vary depending upon the age of your dog. The solutions are mostly measured on a scale, the range of the scale starts from zero and end on 14. Diet is considered alkaline if the pH level is greater than 7. Similarly, the solution is said to be acidic if the pH level measures it below 7.

Aside from specific medicine diets intended to modify a dog's urinary pH level to keep the arrangement of bladder and kidney stones, most financially arranged dog foods will, in general, have acidic pH levels.

What Comprises an Alkaline Diet

A handcrafted alkaline diet is involved in regular raw foods, mainly vegetables. Foods that may build dietary alkaline levels include:

horse feed

apples

bananas

beans

celery

cruciferous vegetables (broccoli and cabbage)

cucurbit vegetables (pumpkins and squash)

potatoes

Regular apple juice vinegar, unsweetened cranberry juice, and vegetable juices can likewise build dietary alkaline levels.

Notwithstanding the vegetables recorded over, your dog's body will benefit from a homemade food diet that incorporates bones and organ and muscle meat. You can enhance the chicken with greens, for example, kale, parsley, romaine, spinach or spirulina green growth, to additionally help its basic level.

The Benefits of Alkaline Water

Alkaline water is considered to have ultra- hydrating characteristics when it is compared to the normal water. This is quite beneficial for the dogs and pets who are or not suffering from any type of disease. The reason lies in that the molecules of water in alkaline water are comparatively smaller, so the absorption power of these alkaline molecules is much greater than the normal water. As this will certainly help pets and even individuals to rehydrate more quickly.

Another good feature of alkaline water is that it boosts immunity. The immune system can help in neutralizing the acidity in the body which may be the result of stress, poor diet, and environmental toxins.

Alkaline water is rich in compounds like calcium and magnesium. These two components are the main source of bone production and development. So, by using alkaline water automatically bones get stronger.

Alkaline water has antioxidants that play a vital role in the growth of damaged cells in the body. Damaged cells when not timely treated cause aging in the individuals.

Another important function of alkaline water is that it brings the acidity at a moderate level. It lowers the quantity of acidity in our body when it crosses the high level. Then again it increases the acidity level when it goes down under a certain level which is injurious to health.

Alkaline water is a considered good when either your pet or any individual is suffered from a chronic disease like cancer or kidney stone etc.

A few organizations are currently touting the health benefits of alkaline ionized water (and the going with water treatment systems) for pets and individuals. This particular water has been credited with enhancing the health of dogs with an assortment of ailments and constant conditions, including:

joint pain

stomach related problems

hip dysplasia

respiratory problems

thyroid issue

kidney stones

What Health Conditions Can Benefits from an Alkaline Diet?

Oxalate stones frame in a dog's urinary tract when his urine is excessively acidic. Making progressively alkaline urine may benefit dogs with these sorts of rocks, and encouraging them an alkaline diet may help roll out this improvement.

The dog that has struvite stones in their urinary tract won't benefit from an alkaline diet as their bodies are now making alkaline urine, which is causing the stones shape. Dogs with these sorts of stones may benefit from other dietary alterations, for example, the momentary utilization of remedy diets or dietary acidifiers to adjust urinary pH levels.

Alkaline diets may likewise not be suggested for some canine kidney problems, which can turn out to be more terrible with an alkaline diet. Dogs that are inclined to visit urinary tract diseases may likewise not benefit from an alkaline diet. Talk about any dietary concerns you have with your veterinarian before changing your pet's food so the person in question can enable you to settle on the best choice for your dog's health.

Why You Should Feed Your Dog an Alkaline Diet?

What Alkaline Means For Your Dog's Health

You may have known about the alkaline diet just like the ideal approach to accomplish prevalent health. This broadly touted eating plan comprises of expending entirely alkaline-promoting foods frequently and disposing of acid forming foods from the diet entirely. That implies maintaining a strategic distance from foods like dairy, grains, caffeine, and liquor in your regular menu. By just eating alkalinizing foods, the pH levels in your body are said to build, which is professed to have stunning benefits, similar to unrivaled assurance against infections and fast weight reduction.

These health benefits aren't merely restricted to people. By lessening the measure of acid forming foods you feed your dog and expanding alkaline-promoting foods, you could be empowering critical enhancements in his general health and prosperity. Alkaline diets for pets are said to diminish the danger of kidney problems, liver problems, and diabetes, among different benefits.

Canine Caviar, the sole alkaline dog food maker, firmly advocates bolstering your pets alkaline-promoting foods for their mind-blowing mending properties. "The alkaline dog food is not the same as some other pet food recipe on the planet." "Having an alkaline based diet help put more oxygen into the blood to permit the DNA's self-recuperation system to work all the more proficiently and adequately."

CHAPTER 15

WHAT IS AN ALKALINE DIET FOR PETS?

By sustaining your dog foods that are over seven on the pH scale, similar to kelp, parsley and horse feed, you are promoting an appropriate pH balance in their body, prompting great health and basic mending. The liquid in a dog's body is somewhat alkaline, and if pH levels of their blood, lymph, and cerebral spinal fluid achieve an acidic level, dogs chance contracting degenerative illness in the tissue.

Canine Caviar utilizes bitter base herbs and fixings in their dog food alongside a novel handling technique to make an alkaline diet. Alkaline-promoting foods are staples in the menus, while acidic foods with a pH lower than 5.2—like hamburger, pork, eggs, wheat, and blueberries—are avoided from their items completely. Adding minerals to the food can likewise build its alkalinity; however, Canine Caviar maintains a strategic distance from this procedure because such a large number of alkaline metals can cause precious stones in the urine, which can prompt kidney stones.

By nourishing Canine Caviar dog food to your dog, their urine will experience a change from acidic urine to somewhat alkaline urine. Canine Caviar will joyfully furnish you with pH test strips for nothing out of pocket so you can observe the difference for yourself.

Benefits of an Alkaline Diet for Dogs

Encouraging dogs entirely alkaline-base diets should put more oxygen in the blood, limit cell degeneration, settle stomach related surprises, and diminish scratching and problem areas. It can likewise reduce the indications of maturing by decreasing anaerobic movement.

You need to give your dog a high caliber alkaline diet, attempt Canine Caviar Limited Ingredient Diet Open Meadow Holistic Entrée Dry Dog Food. This recipe is perfect for dogs with touchy stomach related tracts and is healthfully upgraded to help the advancement of muscles, organs, bones, and teeth. Hormone-, pesticide-and anti-toxin free dried out sheep is the central fixing in this item, and its intriguing nature viably invigorates the immune system in dogs who experience the ill effects of food sensitivities.

For dogs on a wet food diet, there are Canine Caviar 97% Salmon Grain-Free Canned Dog Foods Supplements that can be bolstered as a treat, supplement or as the base of a home-arranged supper. This dog food contains no grains, fillers, including sugar or salt or counterfeit hues or additives, making it an incredible expansion to a strict alkaline dog diet.

Canine Caviar Norwegian Sun-Cured Kelps Dog Food Topper is wealthy in nutrients and minerals, including necessary follow minerals for adjusted development. Kelp advances healthy skin and coat is an incredible assimilation help and helps clean the kidneys, bladder, and uterus. Canine Caviar has exclusive expectations with regards to sourcing their fixings, so you will discover their kelp is of the highest quality, pulled from the coldest waters of Norway. Add this kelp topper to your dog's most loved dish for an overly nutritious dinner that will help decontaminate the blood and upgrade the immune system.

Demonstrate your dog you cherish him with heavenly Canine Caviar Omega 3:6:9 Alkaline Dog Treats, made with premium-quality wild herring and salmon oil to help a gleaming coat and healthy skin. At only three calories for each piece, these alkaline dog treats are extraordinary for preparing, or for those occasions when your great dog merits a reward.

When nourishing your little guy, remember that an appropriate water source is essential for supporting an alkaline diet. Filtered water will, in general, be acidic, while tap water is stacked with dangerous synthetic concoctions. While picking a water hotspot for your pet, search for Ionized Alkaline water, which can expand your dog's resistance to ailment and health difficulties, and help detoxify his indications.

Alkaline Diet for Your Dogs

Expanding your dog's alkaline admission can drastically change their general health. A diet that is wealthy in alkaline settles your pooch's PH levels and enhance their capacity to battle malignant growth causing cells that engenders in over fermented condition.

A natively constructed diet produced using celery, bananas, potatoes, and other characteristic vegetables may expand dietary alkaline levels of your dog. Notwithstanding the greens, you can likewise alkalinize your water by including bentonite clay which is known for having usually high chemical levels. Bentonite clays have as high as 9.0 ph and are a standout amongst the cheapest yet successful characteristic detox apparatuses accessible for the two people and creatures. Collected in the stores close Fort Benton, Wyoming, this matured volcanic clay has been utilized as a detoxification instrument and mending fixing in treating medicinal conditions since pre-notable time. As of not long ago, numerous individuals—and even superstars—are attempting these current natures ponder.

Otherwise called the detoxifying clay, bentonite clay contains a fixed negative charge that can flush out decidedly charged poisons, overwhelming metals, and different polluting influences in our body. Enhanced with different follow components, for example, magnesium, potassium, sodium, iodine, it can likewise be taken inside as a food supplement or mineral swap for the two people and creatures.

CHAPTER 16

THE BEST DIET IF YOU STRUGGLES WITH SILENT ACID REFLUX

There's a particular sort of reflux that is alluded to as "silent" reflux because the individuals who have it don't demonstrate the common symptoms of acid reflux, for example, indigestion. Silent Acid Reflux or Laryngopharyngeal reflux (LPR) is a condition that happens when acid from the stomaches goes up the esophagus the distance to the laryngopharynx in the throat. It is regularly observed in GERD patients, yet may happen alone without GERD.

Symptoms of LPR include:

The vibe of a knot in the throat

Need to make a sound as if to speak much of the time

Gentle dryness

Bodily fluid

Perpetual hack

Trouble gulping

A sore throat

Red or swollen voice box

Hoarseness

A chronic cough or "barking"

Asthma (reactive airways disease)

Noisy breathing or stopping while speaking

Trouble in feeding

Trouble in spitting

Trouble in inhaling food

An unusual increase in weight

Trouble in swallowing something

A feeling of postnasal drip

Excess throat mucus

Contact ulcers

Ear infections

Maybe turning blue

Frequent vomiting

WHO IS MOST LIKELY TO DEVELOP SILENT REFLUX?

Anybody can develop silent reflux, including men, ladies, newborn children, and youngsters. There is some way of life factors that may make grown-ups progressively helpless, including:

Less than stellar eating routine (loads of acidic and spicy foods, an excess of caffeine)

Overeating

Liquor and tobacco misuse

In babies and kids, LPR can develop because of developmental youthfulness of the esophagus.

BEST DIET TO HELP ALLEVIATES SYMPTOMS OF LPR/SILENT REFLUX

Researches have demonstrated that diet assumes a vital job in overseeing silent reflux. Mediterranean foods might be as powerful as proton siphon inhibitors (PPIs) in treating symptoms of acid reflux. Endeavor to treat your symptoms with diet alone, except if advised by your specialist. Medication free treatment may not be appropriate for everybody. Food is medication. What's more, what you put into your body each day assumes a massive job in the state of your health.

If you are suffering from LPR/silent reflux, you should take green leafy vegetables, bananas, celery, melons, and beans. On the other hand, you need to avoid eating spicy fatty and fried foods that may include cheese, garlic, peppermint, chocolate, tomatoes, fruits, and citrus. Furthermore, you need to avoid taking food that contains caffeine, alcohol in particular and carbonated beverages.

People suffering from Laryngopharyngeal reflux (LPR) or silent reflux, it is helpful for them to take the largest meal of the day at midday time or even in the morning as well. They need to avoid taking a large meal at night or evening time. People suffering from Laryngopharyngeal reflux (LPR) or silent reflux probiotic supplement which contains a considerable amount of bacteria that are already available in the body, can ease the symptoms up to a great deal.

WHAT IS A MEDITERRANEAN DIET?

The Mediterranean Diet comes verifiably from the eating propensities and way of life of those living in southern Italy, Greece, Turkey, and Spain. The diet comprises loads of high-fiber fruits and vegetables, quality fats and proteins, and an incidental glass of wine. Because of its many demonstrated health benefits including lessening aggravation, supporting healthy weight, enhancing heart health and diminishing disease chance, the Mediterranean Diet is viewed as one of the healthiest human diets on the planet.

FOODS INCLUDED IN THE MEDITERRANEAN DIET

The most widely recognized, everyday foods of the Mediterranean diet include:

fresh fruits and vegetables (leafy greens, eggplant, cauliflower, artichokes, tomatoes)

olive oil

nuts and seeds (almonds, sesame seeds)

vegetables and beans (lentils, chickpeas)

herbs and flavors (oregano, fennel, rosemary, parsley)

entire grains

wild-got angle/seafood

field raised chicken and eggs

goats drain

fresh water

red wine

A few foods are decently eaten include:

red meat (when week after week)

espresso

tea

kefir and yogurt.

How to Choose High-Quality Olive Oil

Olives have been a staple thing in the Mediterranean locale for more than 5000 years, and those living there devour olive oil as a piece of almost every meal. Not all olive oil is created similarly, be that as it may, and vast numbers of the "olive oil" brands you see on store racks are false impersonations or without their unique supplements. Continuously pick olive oil that is fresh squeezed and extra virgin.

1. Price Points

Good olive oil should cost you less than an amount ranging from $8 to $40. But a truly good olive oil may cost you $25.

2. Taste and Smell Of the Olive Oil

Some people think that the best olive oil has a buttery and sweet taste, but this is not correct. Actually, it tastes in a way that it has been diluted in tasteless vegetable oils. A true olive oil has a pungent smell and a bitter taste. Another way to recognize a good olive oil is that it has the tendency to create a kind of scratch in your throat.

3. Color

Color varies depending upon the ingredients used to prepare it. Olive oil is passed turns golden and finally may go to brownish.

4. Freshness

The beauty of olive oil s that it does not get better after some time, infect it goes it goes worst with the passage of time. The best is to consume it as early as possible.

5. Pure And Light

There is another by which you can make a guess that the olive oil is the best by analyzing it. The real olive oil is pure and light in density, this is for the reason that you can easily use it in baking and deep frying.

6. Cold Pressed

The indication of cold press depicts that while extracting olive from the olives, no heat was applied. Some companies use this technique in order to extract more and more oil from the olives but doing this may well lose the flavor, aroma, and lightness of the oil. Here cold press indicates a temperature of 80.6 Fahrenheit.

PARTHA'S PRESCRIPTIONS FOR SILENT REFLUX

Fiber likewise advances normality of stable discharges and enhances stomach related health. Every day, ladies should expect to expend somewhere around 25 grams of fiber and men, 38 grams.

Eat Small Meals Every 3-4 Hours. Overeating can bother symptoms of reflux since it puts a ton of weight on the stomach and can drive acid up into the esophagus.

Limit Sugar Intake. Most Americans are eating abundant excess sugar. This prompts weight gain and obesity which like this improve the probability of developing silent reflux. The American Heart Association prescribes ladies eat not more than 20 grams of sugar and men eat close to 36 grams.

Caffeine loosens up the esophagus, making it simpler for acid to go up from the stomach and cause reflux symptoms. Spicy foods will, in general, disturb the throat and have found in numerous investigations to bother acid reflux.

If you've made changes in diet and way of life however still can't seem to feel good, it might be an ideal opportunity to counsel with your specialist. Silent Reflux can regularly be a symptom of an increasingly good condition like GERD. Cooperating with a healthcare expert will enable you to settle on the best choices for your one of a kind health need.

CHAPTER 17

ALKALINE DIET FOR GERD

A harsh preference for the back of your mouth or torment in your chest in the wake of eating can be an indication of gastroesophageal reflux disease, otherwise called GERD. Individuals with GERD can utilize drugs for alleviation, however, for some, changes in the diet can help improve a few or the majority of the symptoms. Eating alkaline foods is one methodology that has become a force to be reckoned with as a treatment for GERD.

Alkaline Diet

The basic concept behind Alkaline Diet is to monitor what you are actually putting in your digestive system. The Alkaline diet has been based on one of the ideas that by replacing foods that form acid in your body can play a part in improving your overall health. Not only it can change the pH value in your body but also it helps in the digestion of food as well.

The thought behind the alkaline diet is that as foods are processed, they can create either acidic or chemical substances. Since over the top generation of acid might have the capacity to exasperate gastroesophageal reflux, eating foods that are alkaline - which means they can kill abundance acid - may bring down the measure of acid in the body and help diminish reflux. "Chronicles of Otology, Rhinology, and Laryngology" took a look at the impacts of an alkaline diet on laryngopharyngeal reflux, a type of gastroesophageal reflux disease. This paper found that limiting acidic foods and underscoring alkaline foods decreased the symptoms and clinical indications of this type of GERD, proposing that embracing the alkaline diet can have a unique clinical advantage for individuals with GERD.

Foods to Avoid

You are endeavoring to utilize an alkaline diet to treat GERD, decrease your utilization of acidic foods. For this, you need to reduce the consumption of edible oils that may include olive oil, canola oil, and corn oil as well. Numerous grains are additionally acidic, for example, corn, grain, wheat, moved oats, quinoa, and buckwheat, so most heated products ought to be limited. Numerous creature based proteins, for example, cheddar, meat, and fish will likewise be kept away from, and also peanuts, pecans, walnuts, cashews, and beans.

Proposed Foods

Although you should constrain or evade many foods on the off chance that you are on an alkaline diet, a lot of options are accessible for each meal. Since many grains are acidic, breakfast could comprise of fruits, for example, grapefruit, apples, bananas, grapes, honeydew, oranges, dates, berries and pineapple. Other breakfast options incorporate poached eggs and yogurt. Lunch options combine chicken bosom - which not at all like different meats is alkaline - almonds and curds.

You can take the following foods to manage your symptom of alkaline acidity.

1. Vegetables

Vegetables are thought to have less sugar and fat and certainly help you minimize your stomach acidity. You can take cucumbers, potatoes, leafy greens, broccoli, green beans, asparagus, and bell peppers.

2. Ginger

Ginger has the characteristics of anti-inflammatory and considered as the natural cure for gastrointestinal and heartburn problems. You can easily add sliced ginger and grated ginger in your drinks.

Oatmeal

Oatmeal is a whole grain, breakfast favorite and one of the fantastic sources of fiber. It has the tendency to absorb in the stomach and minimize the symptoms of reflux.

3. Healthy Fats

Looking for the healthy fats, here is the answer to that. You can take walnuts, avocados, sesame oil, flaxseeds, and sunflower oil and so on.

Other Dietary Changes

Notwithstanding eating an alkaline diet, individuals experiencing GERD can roll out different improvements to their diets to limit symptoms. Eating littler meals, for instance, and abstaining from eating before sleep time can decrease GERD symptoms. Certain foods, for example, greasy/seared foods, tomato sauce, chocolate, mint, garlic, and onions can likewise decline GERD.

You are worried about GERD symptoms, converse with your specialist before rolling out any vast improvements to your diet.

There are many experts who are of the view that drinking alkaline water, does not matter whether you purchase it in bottle form or you have created it in your own way from the tap with the help of ionizing purifier, is really healthy to drink it. Now what impact it will make on your body? The answer is simple but clear:

- It slows down your aging process.
- It helps your energy level.
- It helps people who are already suffering from fertility issues.
- It brings your pH at a moderate level.
- It also protects you against lethal diseases like cancer.

IS AN ALKALINE DIET THE SECRET TO CLEARS, GLOWING SKIN?

An excess of acid in our bodies can prompt breakouts. Alkalizing our framework will help quiet our skin so we can avoid skin break out. Our bodies are brilliantly intended to keep a reasonable pH to secure us as well as maintain us process food. At the point when our bodies are in an alkaline state, we can avoid various diseases and keep our bodies stable.

Since delightful skin begins from inside, it makes sense that keeping our inner frameworks stable helps set the establishment for clear, sound skin. Tragically, our cutting-edge diet and way of life advance excessively acid in our bodies. How would we avoid making a lethal domain in our bodies? One means is to eat the right food in the right ways. Doing as such will enable our bodies' pH to remain in the right zone.

The Importance of pH

The term pH (capability of hydrogen) is utilized to allude to how acidic or alkaline an answer depends on the size of 0-14. On that scales, 0 is the most acidic, 14 is the most alkaline, and seven is impartial. The food and drink we consume can either tips that scale toward being increasingly acidic or progressively alkaline.

Furthermore, it is important for your body because pH creates acidity when the bloodstream is too acidic, pH steals the calcium (a substance which is more Alkaline) from the bones in order to bring the acidity a balanced level.

Try not to Consume These 5 Acidic Promoters:

Caffeine

Dairy

Grains

Meat

Handled Food

Avoiding the previously mentioned things is an excellent place to begin; however, we can't stop there. We additionally need to recognize what to add to our diet to enable us to alkalize our bodies and put us on the way to bright, bright skin. It's additionally vital to perceive that the mineral and bicarbonate content of food is similarly as essential as the pH level.

Certain foods like tomatoes or fluids like apple juice vinegar are generally seen as acidic. They are very alkaline in the body because of their mineral and bicarbonate content. What are some different foods and refreshments that assistance alkalize our bodies?

Consume These 5 Alkaline Promoters:

Blueberries

Green smoothie with dim greens like spinach, cucumber, and kale

Homegrown tea

High alkaline ionized water or boiling water with lemon each morning (2 containers w/¼ fresh pressed lemon)

Olive Oil

Not to be neglected is our way of life. What's the purpose of eating the right food if we damage our endeavors with unfortunate propensities?

Avoid These 3 Unhealthy Lifestyle Habits:

Rest shortages

Smoking

Focusing

A simple and successful way to diminish your acid load is to rehearse deep breathing for the day. Remain hydrated and avoid diuretic drinks like espresso and liquor which are diuretics. Diuretics influence you to urinate all the more much of the time and can prompt parchedness because of water problems.

Try not to ransack your cells of precious water. Skin break out prone skin needs all the assistance it can get the opportunity to ward off breakouts and remaining hydrated unquestionably makes a difference. In case you're interested in how alkaline or acidic your body is, there is a simple way to test it from the solace of your own home.

Test Your pH

Measure your pH with litmus paper strips. You can go without stretch purchases litmus paper strips like these that give pH readings that are similarly as exact as the dipsticks specialists use. You can test your saliva or urine. Urine's pH extends differ for the day from acid to alkaline.

Since urine is increasingly acidic in the first part of the day, it is smarter to test the second urine of the day. A good urine run is 6.8-7.5 pH. Saliva's range ought to be from 6.5-7.0.

CHAPTER 18

ALKALINE DIET FOR GOUT

What you eat can influence your well-being somehow, so it isn't stunning to discover that a few foods can likewise improve your feel when you are debilitated or have gout. Study's demonstrate that an alkaline diet for gout is exceptionally successful in diminishing uric acids, which is good to forestall flare-ups and notwithstanding treating gout symptoms.

Cause and Symptoms of Gout

Gout is the rarest type of joint inflammation, and it creates when the level of uric acid in the body is high. Uric acid results in the breakdown of purines that come from the different type of food that we eat in our routine life.

Symptoms of Gout

- **Intense joint pain.** Gout mostly affects the joint of your large toe, but it is not compulsory, this can very much occur in any joint. Other common joints that are affected by the gout are the knee, ankles, wrists, elbows, and fingers. The pain gets severe within four to 12 hours after it starts.

- **Lingering discomfort.** After the most pain subsides, the discomfort in the joints may last from few days to few weeks. Later attacks usually last a touch longer and affect relatively more joints.

- **Inflammation and redness.** The situation becomes critical and abnormalities start appearing. The affected joint or joints become tender, swollen, reddish and warm.

- **Limited Movement.** As gout proceeds from one place to the other, you may not move your joints normally. But when you move them it is most likely that you will feel a lot of pain in these joints.

One of the trigger elements why gout assaults are purine. In this way, any food and drinks that have a high content of purine ought to be avoided, for example, red meat, kidneys, sweetbreads, liver and above all eager to keep the advancement of gout. Purine-rich drinks and foods won't merely expand the likelihood of creating gout, yet also increment the acid level in the body quicker.

Why Alkaline Diet For Gout Recommended

An alkaline diet is extremely powerful in lessening and notwithstanding dispensing with the abundance measure of uric acid in the body. Once you have got control over uric acid, it means you have relieved your gout pain. This is conceivable in light of the facts that an alkaline diet can help keep up the required pH level the body needs to wipe out however much uric acid as could be expected which consequently can help your gout issue.

By eating an alkaline diet, you give your body the most obvious opportunity to dispose of uric acid and not need to manage any gout issues. For some people, it is hard to achieve. But once you achieve it, you feel a lot comfortable than the actual position in which you were.

What Foods Are Good For Alkaline Diet for Gout

- Cantaloupe

- Watermelon

- Papaya

- • Parsley

- • Grapes

- • Mango

- • Cayenne Pepper

- • Kelp

- • Apple

- • Berries

- • Ripe Bananas

- • Avocado

- • Cabbage

- • Sweet corn

- • Pumpkin

- • Garlic

- • Brussels grows

- • Cucumbers

- • Almonds

- • Others

Alkaline Diet For Gout Considerations

There is no uncertainty that gout torment can be challenging to deal with.

Be that as it may, picking an alkaline diet for some is an exceptionally protected a compelling way to stop gout in its tracks. These little changes can go far in helping you avoid those horrendous gout assaults.

Moreover, you can take following alkaline foods that can fight against the gouts:

Celery

Celery is mostly used by the people as a snack, or you can put this into your smoothie. It has got a high amount of potassium that resists in the making of uric acid.

Kale

Kale consists of variety of ingredients like minerals, vitamins and antioxidants.

Cherries

Cherries are full of fiber iron and potassium, a great anti-inflammatory against gout.

As always before rolling out any improvements, it's still a good plan to check with your specialist or therapeutic services supplier before pushing ahead.

CHAPTER 19

THE ALKALINE DIET FOR MEN'S HEALTH

Prevalent among the renowned of this world, alkaline diet, otherwise called the 'alkaline fiery remains diet' or 'alkaline acid diet' gets more fit and counteract extreme medical issues such as diabetes, malignant growth, and joint pain. The establishment of the diet is that a few foods, similar to meat, handled foods, wheat, refined sugar, and, cause your body to create acid, which negatively affects our wellbeing. By killing certain foods, we can assist our body with maintaining its blood pH level. It's a very simple to apply diet which you can do without anyone else.

Likewise with a ton of diets, they are for the most part pursued by women; however, the Alkaline Diet is the same. The inquiry is, how can it influence men? From a man's viewpoint, three things may worry them the most about the Alkaline Diet.

Is Alkaline Diet Suitable for Men?

Men worry they will lose muscle.

Men worry that they should give up a portion of their most loved foods, e.g., meat.

They are stressed they won't have the capacity to consume enough protein.

The above things are a couple of the misguided judgments of the Alkaline Diet; initially, nothing must be given up, as long as everything is taken with some restraint. You can at present have meat and go out to supper; it is additionally conceivable to have bites or treats.

Concerning protein, if you were on a full Alkaline diet, following the recommendations, you would have 60 to 80 grams for each day, while numerous dieticians determine between 30 – 50 grams is perfect for a great many people. You work out in the exercise center, the rule of thumb says you ought to consume around 1 gram for each pound of bodyweight if you need to construct muscles.

Generally, it is observed that men are more prone to eat a temporary diet. But here the case is totally different, the alkaline diet is considered to be a long time strategy. The question is why to take alkaline diet for a longer period of time. The answer is simple as the alkaline diet brings small or little changes over the period of time which will result in a much happier and healthier lifestyle.

If you pursue the Alkaline Diet 20/80 rule, muscle problems isn't an issue, because of the number of nutrients, protein, and good fats.

Along these lines, to expose the three stresses is simple.

One of the principle reasons individuals quit any diet is they endeavor to be close immaculate; however, this prompts dissatisfaction with an inclination to stop as they race into it and feel denied.

Numerous men have a look at the expression, "healthy eating" and connect it with a transitory diet. In reality, following the Alkaline Diet is a long-term methodology that will make little changes after some time, and this will lead you into a lot more beneficial way of life.

By its exceptional nature, practice is an acid shaping movement, where part of the recuperation procedure is the place the body attempts to beat the arrangement of acids. This is the place the Alkaline Diet is particularly valuable, as individuals have lost a touch of their standard capacity to consume fat because of a high acid shaping diet. This is especially valid with foods that contain gluten. Presently when you are following the Alkaline Diet, the body can make full utilization of the pancreas, where the body would now be able to get to its fat stores which profoundly affect stamina and perseverance.

For muscle working, there is presently an entirely fuelled diet that is high in cancer prevention agents, and which scrubs and manufacture new oxygen-rich platelets. Additionally, there is adequate protein, healthy fats, and oils and plentiful measures of hydration accessible, so it is likewise profoundly versatile to fit in with any training project you might pursue.

It has dependably appeared, that eating a high amount of nutrient-rich foods has dependably been good for the body, particularly on the off chance that you are into training or sports a great deal. Stomach related problems turn into a relic of days gone by, and poorly tempered entrail disorder or stomach issues wind up facilitated.

As most men will in general like eating meat, they ought to enhance their quality. Along these lines, when shopping, it is much improved to pick the unfenced, field-raised or grass bolstered meats. It might prompt a somewhat little bit; however, it will be increasingly nutrient rich if it originates from a progressively maintainable source and will contain substantially more flavor. Not just this, the creatures won't have been treated with anti-infection agents or steroids as occurs with mass cultivated beings.

Which Food Should You Eat More According to The Alkaline Diet?

Essential Foods

The alkaline diet underlines alkaline foods, for example, vegetables, products of the entire soil grains.

Proteins

Protein is one of the most important components in your body. The best function of protein is that it repairs and builds tissues in your body.

For the best impact, it is best to make beyond any doubt the protein you eat originates from an assortment of sources as opposed to only one source. Rather than 1 or 2 servings of meat, your protein can be spread over other alkaline-shaping foods like verdant greens, vegetables, nuts and seeds and so forth., and if this is as yet not adequate while you are training, you can likewise include a scoop of grew, alkaline non-dairy protein powder. It is fitting to give the falsely seasoned and synthetic based ones a miss.

The grew dark colored rice protein powders contain protein levels of around 25-30 grams for each glass, and whenever blended with non-dairy drain, the standard will be up to 35 grams of protein for every drink.

Natural products

Bananas, Berries, Apples, Pineapple, Grapes, Lemons (acidic ordinarily, however, changes over to high alkaline in the body, and Melons (particularly Watermelons).

Vegetables

Kale, Spinach, Cucumber, Cauliflower, Broccoli.

The majority of the above foods are pressed brimming with nutrients and nutrients and give the appropriate measure of sugars and protein.

It might appear eating like these can be a colossal errand, particularly the measure of spinach and kale that is required. The Alkaline Diet recommends an extent of your foods ought to be eaten uncooked, accordingly protecting any nutrients that are lost while cooking. In this way, these can be gotten through a smoothie, and there are a few blenders available now, that not at all like a juicer, utilize the skins and stalks of specific foods grown from the ground as a feature of the drink. The blender separates everything to the micronutrient level and into a consistency which is drinkable and exceptionally reviving.

You can make this a little stride further, and add nuts or seeds to the blender. At the point when these get separated, you have superfoods in a glass, loaded with proteins and nutrients, and considerably more advantageous for devouring whenever of the day. Either for breakfast or after a good exercise.

Supplements

There are an extensive variety of supplements accessible for men, mainly if they are very dynamic or overwhelming exercise center goers. It is increasingly fitting to adhere to the more normal choices if conceivable - as opposed to the human-made variations. By keeping this straight, you are adding to every one of the nutrients from the foods instead of supplanting them with pills or drinks.

Greens

Powdered green drinks are an excellent expansion to your diet, and you can have either unadulterated wheatgrass or a grass blends. The grass blend is the betters of the two, while the untouched grass is the more financially savvy choice.

Minerals and Salts

As support against the high acid arrangement, you can take alkaline salts or supplements that incorporate magnesium, calcium, potassium, and sodium which are suitable for this. If you can't find an excellent soluble salt supplement, find a good multi mineral and take with a teaspoon of sodium bicarbonate, in a glass of water once every day.

Alcohol

As was recently mentioned, all is well with some restraint. Alcohol is the equivalent, on the off chance that you make informed choices of when it is worth having a drink, at that point, you will find that as a rule, you will need to make the correct decision. So at last, this informed choice will enable you to get the equalization right in your way of life. You will likewise come to realize this is a night off from your routine, and the next day you will pay it back with your green smoothies and vegetables. Endeavor to confine your admission, since you are in charge here.

When you have been following the alkaline diet for some time, you will find you have turned out to be self-directing your admission, as your objectives of being fit and healthy are in sight. You can perceive what is attainable and adhere to a suitable arrangement, as long as possible. You have the right to be healthy.

ALKALINE DIETS AND PREGNANCY: FROM FERTILITY TO A BLISSFUL PREGNANCY

Truly outstanding and superb experience a lady can ever have is the demonstration of bringing a youngster into this world. The energy and happiness that has been appended to it are very boundless, and it accompanies the unfathomed want to secure, support and keeping the baby healthy. We will take considerations at basic diet and pregnancy, how a high pH diet helps the health of a pregnant lady emphatically. Like we as a whole know, fertility assume an outstanding job in pregnancy. This is a long book, tailing it a tiny bit at a time will give a more precise understanding why keeping up a high pH (antacid) diet is beneficial for fertility and having an ecstatic pregnancy.

Eating and drinking soluble foods and water isn't only the best thing you can improve the situation the health of your baby, but at the same time is an extraordinary method to lighten a portion of the side effect of being pregnant.

For a smoother understanding, let us address this dialog under the accompanying sub-headings:

1. 1. The effect of acidic pH on ladies' fertility

2. 2. Alkalinity and getting pregnant

3. 3. Keeping a joyful pregnancy

4.   So, you should proceed!

The effect of acidic pH on ladies' fertility

The pH of the vagina is somewhat unique about that of the body since menstrual cycles and hormones have influenced it. Ordinary pH of the vagina is between the scope of 3.8 to 4.5. Be that as it may, amid ovulation, the pH of the vagina ought to be somewhere around 7 to 14. This pH goes considered exceptionally antacid, and it is non-dangerous to sperm.

How might you decide the pH of your vagina?

Different packs have been sold in drug stores and medication stores that you can without much of a stretch use in deciding the pH of your vagina. It includes applying the test strips to the internal mass of your vagina for a few minutes, bring it out, at that point look at the shading change on the piece with a shading coded screen graph to decide your vaginal pH.

If your pH is excessively acidic (which means it is disagreeable for sperms), you should eat basic foods or foods that can diminish the acidic nature. There are numerous healthy antacid foods out there, for example, beans, vegetables, grains, and healthy omega oils. Fresh leafy foods, albeit acidic in raw structures yet they alkalinity affect the body. Sugar, in the long run, transforms into acid inside the body, subsequently ought to be extraordinarily evaded.

In the end in the wake of testing your vaginal pH and you find that it is excessively acidic, the best counsel is to counsel your doctor.

Alkalinity and getting pregnant

Too much quantity of acidity in the body can also affect the fertility. Usually, it is observed that sperms like to live in a slightly alkaline environment. On the other hand, too much quantity of acidity also affects the women with endometriosis, sometimes taking the situation to a worse level.

Guaranteeing that the body is kept up by having the best possible alkalinity is rapidly turning into a vital factor that ladies look for to build their odds of getting pregnant.

For what reason is alkalinity so critical in getting pregnant?

Indeed, we have examined it as of now. However, you see that the pH of the body is a smidgen on the primary side, which is around 7.5 out of a conceivable 14 which proposes that your body's normal state is only a minor piece towards being soluble.

What does terrible pH mean?

At the point when the body gathers a great deal of acidic substance in them, it can in the result to a ton of health issues. Corrosiveness can cause problems like urinary tract contaminations, vaginal diseases, yeast contaminations, menstrual challenges, parasitic, and even infertility. Sperm usually cherishes an antacid situation, so when the diet and ways of life of a lady prompts a progressively acidic condition, it tends to be very hard to get pregnant. An acidic domain inside the vagina can make the cervical bodily fluid murder the sperms. This is indeed not what a lady planning to get pregnant will incline toward.

Keeping a euphoric pregnancy

Many side effects are engaged with being pregnant. From heart consume and morning sickness to swollen feet and pregnancy brain. Although the vast majority of these side effects are healthy, the vast majority don't understand that they can be avoided. They happen because of being got dried out and absence of soluble minerals. So a straightforward answer for this is everyday drinking of soluble water.

Studies have uncovered that the body pH of eager mothers drops towards being acidic amid pregnancy. There are two noteworthy purposes behind this:

1. 1. A developing baby requires antacid minerals which it gets from the mother's body. This need will debase the mother's antacid store and drops her pH to being acidic, rather than necessary.
2. 2. As the hatchling develops, it assimilates supplements from the umbilical string, and once these minerals have been consumed, they make acidic squanders which assembles in the placenta. Since the veins of the mother aren't associated with that of the hatchling, her thread can't do the waste, their creation the causticity to gathers in her body.

Drinking mineralized and soluble water previously, amid and after pregnancy helps in enhancing the mother's body, setting it up to manage all the change related to being pregnant.

Presently given us a chance to take a look at the side effects of being pregnant and how soluble water would be able to kill them and make life ecstatic.

1. Morning sickness

Morning sickness is considered not harmful either for the baby or for the mother in general. According to research, about 50% of pregnant ladies do experience morning sickness. Several doctors suggest to their patients that morning sickness is not a bad thing actually. If you experience morning sickness, it means the placenta is increasing most probably in the right direction.

Morning sickness is caused by a sudden adjustment in the body's pH, and this regularly happens when the embryo requires soluble minerals from the mother's body, debasing the mother's antacid stores. By drinking a more significant amount of soluble water, the agency will have enough minerals for both the mother and he baby, with the goal that the shape of the mother won't move to a sudden acidic state, counteracting morning sickness.

What to do in Morning Sickness

- You need to take small meals many times a day.
- You need to drink fluids 1 or half an hour before or after the meal but remember not during the meal.
- Keep taking fluids after intervals so that you do not get dehydrated.
- Eat whatever you like to eat and whenever you want to eat.
- Keep the windows open.
- If odor bothers you then keep the fan on constantly.
- Avoid going to warm places.
- Sniff sour things like ginger, lemon or eat a lot of watermelons.
- Keep an alkaline potato chip bag with you.

- Have a decent walk after every meal

- Try to take a lot of rest in the day.

- Try to have plenty of sleep in the day and also in the night.

What not to do

- Do not lie after eating a meal.

- Try not to skip a meal.

- Do not keep this situation as untreated.

- Try not to eat spicy food or try not to cook anything.

2. Swollen hands and feet

This is for the most part essential in the third trimester, and water maintenance is an indication of lack of hydration. At this stage, the pregnant mother should expand her admission of water to make up for the additional weight gain for the baby. Water maintenance happens when the body attempts to clutch however much water as could be expected, in the mission of not having enough. Appropriate hydration is vital to this circumstance.

3. Lower back torment

Lower back agony is additionally an indication of parchedness. It is caused because of expanded weight and weight from the uterus, and it is typically seen in the second and third trimesters. The plates pad the vertebrate of the spinal harmony, expect water to anticipate rubbing, which prompts aggravation, causing the back agony. Soluble water contains calcium, which reinforces the muscles and bones. Consequently, essential water is more effective than tap water.

4. Acid reflux and heartburn

The hormones that loosen up muscles amid pregnancy (progesterone) additionally loosens up the stomach valve that keeps corrosive out of the throat. The embryo swarms the stomach and power corrosive into the throat, bringing about a terrible circumstance. Regular drinking of essential water avoids acid refluxes and heartburn.

5. Clogging

The significant reason for obstruction is the absence of adequate water consumption. Drinking essential water will help in greasing up the digestive system and flush out squanders.

6. Dry and irritated skin

The human body is comprised of 70% of water, and the skin is the biggest organ in the human body. Amid pregnancy, the surface extends, and on the off chance that it isn't appropriately hydrated, it will end up dry and bothersome.

7. Weariness

Because of expansion in weight and hormones, and absence of value rest, weariness and low energy levels are extremely regular amid pregnancy. Soluble water does not just hydrates the body, is additionally helps minerals in the body. These two things will streamline the body capacity and increment the energy levels.

8. Poor rest

A considerable lot of these side effects dependably keep a pregnant mother up around evening time. Drinking mineralized and antacid water mitigates the general distress that thwarts a peaceful rest.

9. Pregnancy brain

Magnesium, one of the minerals in antacid water, have been appeared to enhance memory. Drinking soluble water will influence the brain to be completely hydrated, to decrease carelessness and enables the brain to work ideally.

10. By and large health

Amid pregnancy, it is imperative to settle on choices that will keep up the health of the mother and the baby. Customary drinking of antacid water will expand the body's pH which will fortify each component of the body, making it as healthy as could reasonably be expected.

Conclusion

The Alkaline Life Diet holds great importance in sustaining your overall health balance. This diet is mainly comprised of fresh fruits and vegetables. Making these leafy greens a big chunk of your diet can help you restore your pH balance. Whereas, the acidic diet when taken in large amounts can be fatal. It's important for all of us to keep an 80/20 alkaline to the acidic ratio in order for us to live a long and healthy life. Because of our busy and fast pace life, many people are eating these "convenience" foods in their daily diet. During this time, diseases are also increasing, and new diseases are manifesting every year.

At the end of the day your health is your wealth and extreme efforts should made to maintain it in order to really LIVE YOUR BEST LIFE.

The facts confirm that numerous individuals who have shifted to an alkaline diet plant based diet observed noteworthy health improvements. With the prevalence of numerous diseases, it is getting very important for every individual to embark on an alkaline life diet. This book is written for all those who need help pertaining to the incorporation of an alkalizing diet in their life. This book was written to help all those who feel at a loss while searching for ways to introduce alkaline foods into their diets. I would like to thank everyone for allowing me to teach you about the health benefits of having an alkaline body. It's been a blessing for me to be granted the ability to help everybody out there looking to live there best life by improving their overall health. Please take a look at the Alkaline Life Diet website for more books in the

ALKALINE DIET SERIES ---->> https://the-alkaline-life-diet.myshopify.com THANK YOU TO ALL & GOD BLESS EVERYONE

www.ingramcontent.com/pod-product-compliance
Lightning Source LLC
Chambersburg PA
CBHW061353250726

48657CB00004B/1472